Causes of Weight Gain in EDS

Lynne D M Noble

All rights reserved. No part of this publication may be reproduced, stored in a retrieval system or transmitted in any form or by any means, without prior permission in writing of the author Lynne D M Noble, or as expressly agreed by law, or under terms agreed with the appropriate reprographics right organisation.

You must not circulate this book in any other binding or cover and you must impose the same condition on any acquirer.

Independently published 2020

About the Author

Lynne Noble was born in 1953 in Huddersfield, West Yorkshire. From a very early age, Lynne showed an interest in nutrition and genetics avidly reading any books that she could get her hands on at the time.

Initially, Lynne studied orthopaedics but events led her to work with the elderly mentally infirm. Here, her interest in neurodegenerative disorders and pain syndromes developed.

Lynne undertook rigorous programmes of study, completing her Cert Ed., (FE) BSc (Hons) and Adv. Dip Education simultaneously before moving onto her M.Ed.

From there she took further demanding programmes in Human Nutrition, Pharmacology, Neuroscience, Genetics and Immunology. During this time, she was given many prestigious awards for her academic work. It was noted then that Lynne was not afraid of tackling difficult subjects.

She began her law degree but ill health prevented her from pursuing this. However, in this time, she moved from being a foster parent to adoptive parent.

She has been instrumental in setting up projects in the community for disadvantaged groups.

She is a member of the Guild of Health Writers.

Now retired, she lives with her husband in a historic Georgian riverside town in the West Midlands. She enjoys gardening, watching her husband bowling and researching.

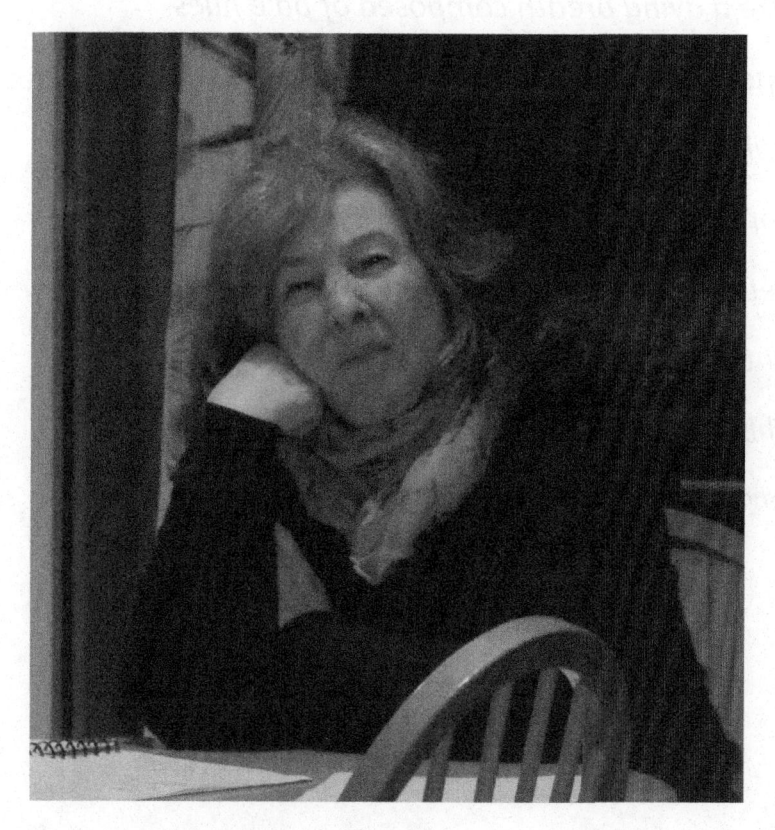

Author Lynne Noble at home

https://quintessentiallylynne.weebly.com/nutritional-medicine.html

Fragility wraps itself around her

Like a dying breath composed of pale hues

And longing that the time of departure

Will be stayed, yet knowing it will not.

For life is ever short,

Yet the pain of life much longer

But still, tis sweet

This life, made sweeter by its brevity.

Lynne D M Noble 2018

Contents

Preface	vii
A personal Anecdote	1
Double trouble – heat oedema and thin veins	8
Lymphoedema	25
Allergies, angieoedema and mast cell activation disorder	35
Long term protein deficiency	57
Table of Medications causing weight gain	65
Two dietary changes to consider	72
Vitamin D deficiency and weight gain	80
Progesterone deficiency	86
Inflammation	92
Trace elements	93
Brown fat, white fat	105
Final word	113

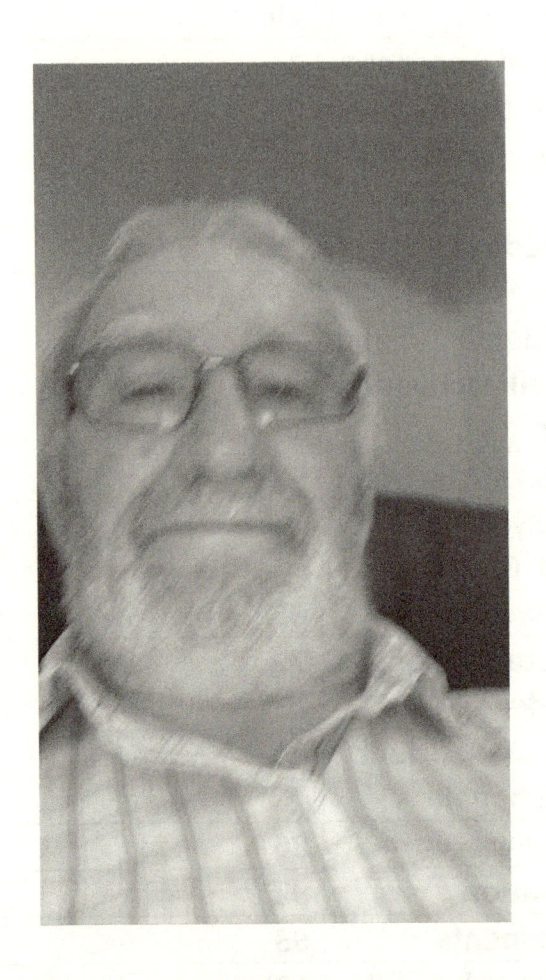

This book is dedicated to my cousin

Bob James

Who inspired me to write this book

Preface

EDS is a systemic disorder and, as such, the manifestations of this syndrome in all its forms are diverse. Those who have EDS will no doubt be aware of painful joints, easy bruising, gastroparesis to name but a few. Indeed, these will be included among the many disparate symptoms of EDS that make this condition so difficult to diagnose in the first place.

However, during my research, I have come across heart-rending tales from EDSers' who have unwanted weight changes. Some have put on weight and failed to lose it in spite of disciplined dieting. Coping with a debilitating condition is hard enough. Often a little retail therapy can restore mood but changes in body mass are hard for most people to cope with at the best of times. A reminder that you don't look as you would like, in spite of intensive efforts, may actually worsen self-esteem.

Many health professionals fail to understand why these changes occur. How often have I heard patients say that they have felt belittled and angered by health professionals who believe an increase in body mass is solely down to poor food choices. In EDS - as in other conditions- this may not be the case, at all. Nevertheless, until patients are confident in understanding the reasons why these changes may occur, they cannot discuss with - and inform - their caregivers with any assured competence that it is not poor food choices that are contributing to increased body mass.

The Body Mass Index (BMI) is not an accurate measure for many people. Those who are older, taller, shorter or more muscular than the 'average' person will find that the BMI does not accurately place an individual in the correct category. Thus many healthy people are pronounced an unhealthy weight. Therefore, EDSer's may be carrying normal fat but still rate high on the BMI scale.

Further, the BMI cannot tell you where you are **carrying** any extra fat. The fat carried around the abdomen is potentially far more hazardous than that found on the hips. Abdominal fat – found in apple shaped people pumps out inflammatory chemicals. It is found in conditions such as metabolic syndrome and diabetes.

Therefore, those with EDS need to be wise on a number of levels if they are firstly to evaluate the reason for their weight gain and secondly, consider if it is damaging to health.

In contrast, many EDSers' lose concerning amounts of weight. There are many reasons for this and some of these will be explored in this book. However, it is fairly safe to say that even though genetics may provide a susceptibility to this condition and to a set of specific symptoms, environmental factors have the deciding say in whether and how these symptoms are manifested.

There is an art to learning how to structure your environment so that it works for you. Many people with chronic conditions have to do this. Within a short time, any changes to lifestyle become the norm.

This is no less important a concept when it comes to controlling unwanted weight changes.

Alongside these extra measures that you may have to instigate, it is imperative that an EDSer incorporates into their diet meals that provide the nutrients necessary to build good connective tissue. All the information that you need can be found in the book entitled

The EDS and Hypermobility Syndrome Diet

By Lynne D M Noble

This diet is not a difficult one to follow at all. Ease of adherence is a necessity if individuals are to keep to it and make it a permanent part of their lives.

Eventually, it will become second nature to prepare meals that support the synthesis of good connective tissue. This may resolve many of the issues that are part and parcel of living with connective tissue disorders, anyway.

If the weight issues are not resolved then we need to look a little further at the possible reasons and, just as importantly, responses to these.

This seems a good point to turn our attention to the main part of the book. As weight gain appears to concern people more than weight loss, we will start the book by looking at this subject first. A personal anecdote would not come amiss in this section.

A Personal Anecdote

I had always been a super busy person. I worked in health and education while furthering my academic potential and raising three children, often singlehandedly.

Interspersed with this whirlwind life, I suffered numerous sprains and subluxations, jaw problems, gastroparesis, ongoing pain, sciatica (big time) allergies, PoTS to name but a few.

I became on good terms with many of the medical staff at the local hospital. Some were kind and recognised that the swollen joints and ongoing pain were due to an underlying disorder that hadn't yet been named. Others could be quite scathing and hurtful. I am not a person given to tears but comments along the lines that I was making it all up, did hurt.

I coped – most times – with all this. I learned to edge along, with my back against the wall, when my tendons in my ankles were inflamed and painful. I learned that walking sideways relieved the pain a little. Sure, it looked funny when I was out, but it did get me around.

I did have a few bouts when I would be ambling along enjoying the sunshine and then find that suddenly .. splat ..... I would find myself flat on my face. My ankle tendons would just decide not to support me anymore. Sometimes, I would damage my wrist or shoulders and that would be another few months, or even years before movement and strength would be restored.

There are some good points about EDS. I know some of you, on reading this, will probably think that I have taken leave of my senses but I can assure you that I haven't. When I go to the podiatrist, she will comment on my beautiful skin. Apparently, I have the best feet and legs ever. They are not calloused or wrinkled, they are smooth and soft.

'What do you put on your skin?' my chiropodist will ask me. 'People half your age, don't have skin anywhere near as good as this. Even my skin is not as good and I am a podiatrist and know how to care for my feet and legs.'

I tell her that I don't put anything on it and that is the truth. People with EDS often have a smooth, velvet like skin. Wrinkles generally are few and far between.

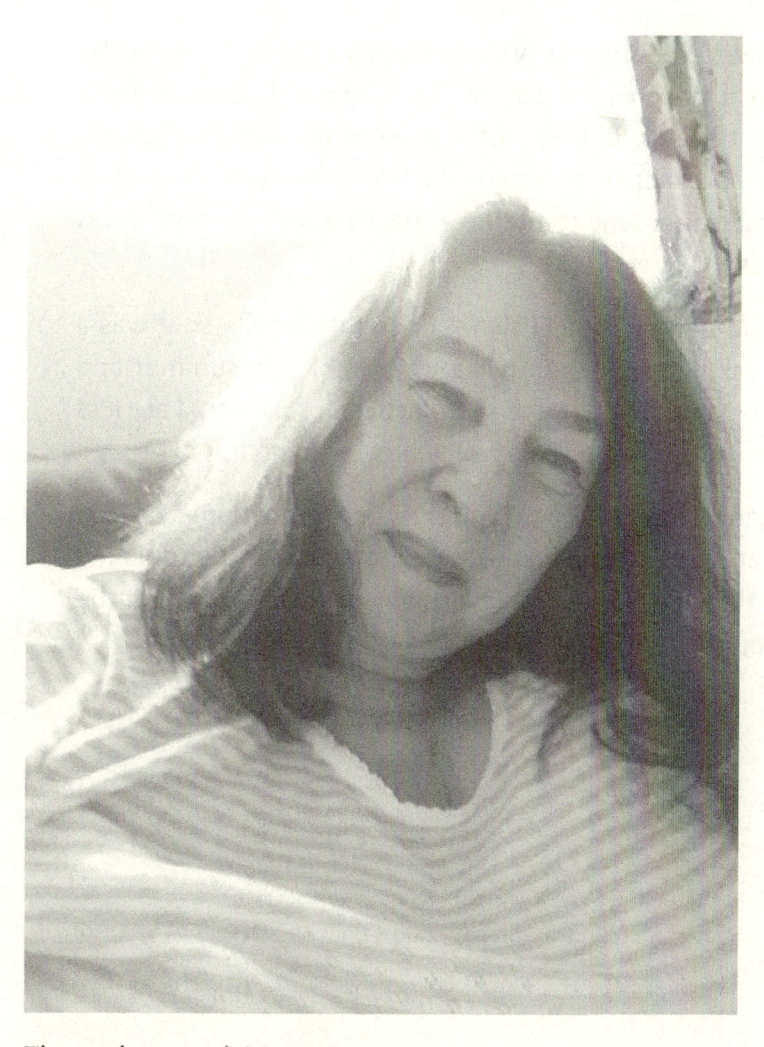

The author aged 66 years.

However, I cannot say there are many advantages to EDS but it becomes a way of life. I adapted. Nevertheless, what I really did find difficult were the weight changes. To be exact, the comments from health professionals who wanted me to fit into a specific range for body mass index.

I had been naturally slim – or so I thought – so it was a shock when I began piling on weight one summer and could not shift it. I was more active in summer. I ate less due to the heat. I was never good with heat.

I had my annual check with the nurse practitioner. I knew that my one swollen ankle and foot accounted for some of the weight gain but it certainly did not account for the majority of it.

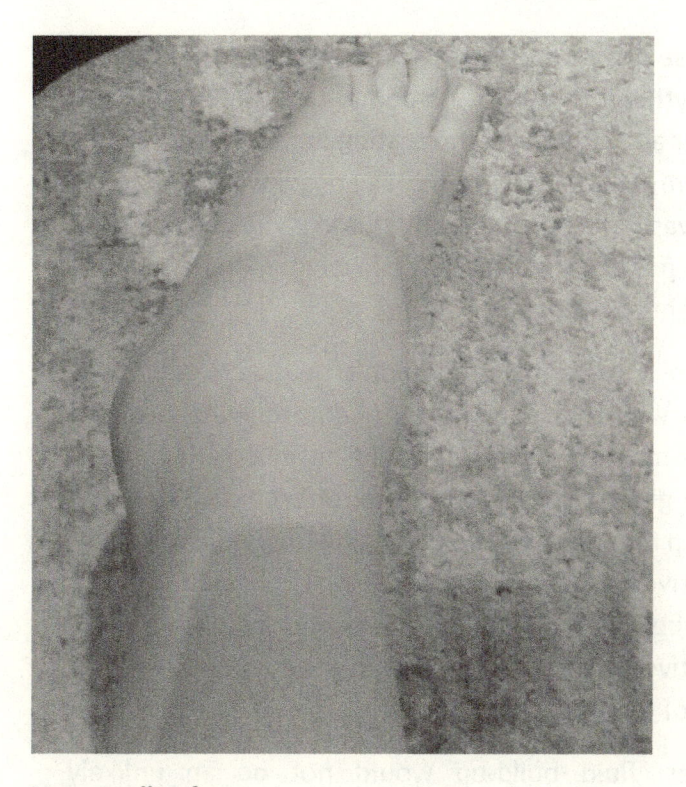

Very swollen foot

The normal contours of my body had disappeared entirely. I was hardly peeing but tests showed that my kidneys and heart health were fine.

In some desperation, I tried the protein shakes that are guaranteed to help you lose weight. I was disciplined but I continued to put weight on.

The nurse practitioner by this point was slightly bemused by everything. There was no point in me reiterating over and over again that I was not eating unhealthily or blindly serving myself extra portions. The proof was there for all to see wasn't it. Too many calories in is the only way that you can put on large amounts of weight? That's what we are taught to believe.

Well, no it isn't and it shouldn't be. There are many reasons why that extra weight- according to the BMI charts - may not be fat. It could be muscle but this is unlikely given that great physical effort – the sort that builds up muscle – may be damaging to people with poor connective tissue. At the very least, physical exercise should be taken slowly and certainly not until a good connective tissue diet has been followed rigorously for a couple of months.

However, fluid build-up would not be an unlikely explanation for weight gain for those with EDS, especially - but not confined to - during warmer months.

Half way through September, I noticed that my weight was going down. At this point I had given up on any calorie restriction. I wasn't motivated when I wasn't getting any positive results. I was exercising the same and eating healthily. Every morning I stepped on the scales and found I had lost a little more.

I changed the battery. I stepped on and off them a few times. I bought new scales but his phenomenon continued until I could get right back into my pre-summer clothing without any problems whatsoever.

At first I thought that it was some weird fluke but this same pattern continued year in and year out. I changed the month of my annual check-up because the weight changes were so great. At least that saved me from having to explain why I was gaining weight rapidly when I was stating that my diet was healthy.

At that point I had changed GP's. I had a lovely nurse practitioner who never criticised. When I relayed how my weight fluctuated according to the seasons, she just smiled.

'You're a conundrum, Lynne, she said, 'but that doesn't mean that it isn't happening.'

I had heard of this phenomenon in other EDSer's so it was about time I put my investigative hat on and begin to dig a little deeper.

Double Trouble – heat oedema and thin veins

Heat oedema is a very common complaint especially among older people where the ageing process has thinned connective tissue. In people with EDS, the thinning of tiny blood vessels will be part and parcel of living with a disorder where collagen is poorly formed. Heat oedema may affect EDSers at a young age.

Oedema happens when capillaries leak fluid into the surrounding tissue. Capillaries are tiny blood vessels that link the arterioles and venules.

Arterioles are the blood vessels that supply blood – containing oxygen and nutrients - to the capillary beds. The capillary beds exchange these for waste products and return them to the venules.

Venules feed into veins which will ultimately return the blood back to the heart.

When the capillaries leak fluid it builds up in nearby tissues. Individuals with EDS have particularly thin blood vessel walls. Fluid is able to pass much more easily through them into the surrounding tissue. This fluid can cause quite a dramatic weight gain over a short period of time.

Individuals with heat oedema can drink good quantities of fluid but find that they are not urinating much. You will have a good idea that heat oedema is a cause of weight gain if you tend to swell in hot weather and urine input appears much greater than output.

Of course there may be other reasons such as kidney or heart problems but most health professionals like to look at the most likely causes first.

The resultant swelling is painful. After all, the tissues are distended. They are not meant to be plumped up unnaturally with fluid that ordinarily would remain inside blood vessels.

Just as heat may cause leaky vessels, reducing the ambient temperature can reverse the process. I have found that air conditioning is a necessity, not a luxury, for people with heat related weight gain.

I have recently moved into an apartment. It did not have air conditioning and subsequent enquiries unfortunately confirmed that installation of a new system would not be possible given its location.

This coincided with a heat wave. Our south facing picture window had a lovely view but it magnified the heat. My abdomen expanded visibly. I could not stand to wash up because if my abdomen pressed against the unit edge it was too painful.

Clearly other measures had to be taken.

Initially, I placed a towel on my abdomen and placed a bag of frozen cauliflower on top of it. After fifteen minutes I could hear gentle gurgling sounds. Fluid was moving. In the morning, when I weighed myself, I found that I had lost one kilogram.

Clearly, keeping cool is a necessity. In the absence of air con, I have had to employ a number of ways to prevent capillary leakage.

A fan does not generally low the ambient temperature. It only pushes the air around but generally makes you more comfortable by evaporating sweat.

A fan can be made into a mini cooler by standing two litre bottles of frozen water in front of it The air that blows is very cooling and refreshing. It takes a fair amount of time for the bottles of frozen water to melt by which time there are already another couple of bottles of water in the process of being frozen ready to replace them.

I also wring out towels soaked in water. If I place them in the refrigerator for half an hour or so, they are nice and cool. I will place them on a swollen area and direct the fan over them. I only need to do this once or twice daily, in the warmer months, for it to be effective. It is a small price to pay to be comfortable.

Varicose veins also promote fluid retention in the legs. In a similar way to capillary leakage, varicose veins leak fluid into the surrounding tissue. While heat may contribute to this process, it is poor valve function that ultimately promotes the problem.

Individuals with EDS are prone to varicose veins from an early age. Legs can become very heavy with fluid. The fluid often pools in the lower legs and ankles. When this happens a number of problems may occur,

- some of the feeling in the feet may be lost.
- As the feet are unusually heavy there is a greater risk of tripping
- Footwear may not fit

Fluid accumulation in the legs and feet can add quite a few pounds to your weight. The accepted treatments for peripheral oedema due to varicose veins are:

- Support stockings
- Raising the legs above the level of the heart whenever possible
- Diuretics*
- Reduce salt in the diet as this attracts fluid

Herbal remedies are unlikely to be effective if the cause is due to poor formation of connective tissue. However, there is no harm in trying some of the more effective remedies on the market to see if they help.

*A word of caution about diuretics. Diuretics are very effective at removing fluid but their side effects can worsen other symptoms of EDS.

Furosemide, a popular diuretic for example, can worsen swallowing problems and impair gastric motility. As these tend to be common – and distressing - problems in those with some types of EDS, then solving one set of problems at the expense of others is not a wise move.

Diuretics tend to remove potassium and magnesium in urine. Magnesium has many functions one of which includes regulating water balance in the body. Low magnesium levels can impact negatively on many of the body's systems. Low magnesium levels can be responsible for

- Gastroparesis
- Water retention
- Poor sleep quality
- Anxiety and depression
- Osteoporosis
- Pain
- High blood pressure
- High blood sugar levels

When a magnesium deficiency occurs the levels of fatty acids are reduced. Skin becomes less elastic and prone to wrinkling.

If you find that the only way forward for you is to use diuretics, then make sure that you take a magnesium supplement. Supplements of 500mg should be adequate.

Potassium – a macro-mineral - is also vital for the smooth running of the body's systems. In fact, it helps prevent excess fluid retention by regulating fluids around your cells. It seems particularly foolish to take diuretics which are going to promote the very problem that you are taking them for in the first place.

In the first instance, increasing foods that contain potassium should be considered. Good sources of foods containing potassium are:

- Potatoes
- Mushrooms
- Bananas
- Dark leafy greens
- Squash
- Tomato juice
- beans

In addition, potassium helps boost the metabolism. Too little potassium can result in confusion, tiredness and muscle aches.

Potassium is required to process iron in the body efficiently and it is needed to help build muscle. Muscle tissue helps to burn calories. Hypokalaemia, the medical term for low potassium levels, may result in

- gastroparesis
- low blood pressure and a PoTS like syndrome
- shortness of breath
- mineral deficiencies

Potassium levels are also intimately connected with the amount of muscle mass an individual has. [1]Studies have shown that potassium values decrease with age and that this is linked to a decrease in muscle mass.

Studies have even shown that abdominal obesity results in hypokalaemia.[2] However, the reverse is also true.

High doses of Furosemide can also affect levels of thyroid hormones. Low levels of thyroid hormones will inevitably cause weight gain.

---

[1] Y.L. Cheng, A.W. Yu, in Encyclopedia of Food Sciences and Nutrition (Second Edition), 2003
[2] https://onlinelibrary.wiley.com/doi/pdf/10.1111/j.1751-7176.2008.07817.x

Therefore, in cases of oedema where tests have ruled out other conditions which may contribute to it, the first port of call should not be diuretics. If the oedema is due to heat, then adjust your environment so that it is cooler.

If a high salt diet is exacerbating problems, then go on a low salt diet.

If peripheral oedema is a problem, then incorporate the responses that I have already mentioned.

In some cases, you may have to incorporate all of the responses.

If diuretics are prescribed, then there are potassium sparing diuretics. You may have to ask for these. Health professionals generally start off with the cheapest prescription drug and work their way up a list of drugs that can treat specific conditions. You may not, initially, get the best treatment for a condition.

These potassium sparing diuretics are not magnesium sparing either so you will still have to address and magnesium deficit.

Magnesium levels are not checked for unless there are signs of a specific problem such as kidney trouble or diabetes.

Potassium levels are generally easier to test for. However, although diuretics are quite commonly prescribed, and for long periods, I have never known anyone have routine checks to ascertain what their potassium levels are after they have use diuretics for a short while.

Potassium is one of the nutritional substances that are not generally supplemented. This is because elevated levels can quickly cause problems just as low levels can.

The way forward is to eat a wide variety of potassium containing foods rather than take a supplement.

Lipoedema and Lymphoedema

The distinction between lipoedema and lymphoedema is fairly straightforward. Lipoedema is a chronic condition where there is an abnormal build-up of fat cells.

These fat cells are generally deposited in the legs and buttocks although the arms may be involved.

Women are generally affected, men only rarely.

Lipoedema fat was initially described in the 1940's by Drs Allen and Hines. They referred to it as

Abnormally poor resistance to the passage of fluid into the tissue from the blood thus permitting oedema to occur.

This observation neatly ties lipoedema as a connective tissue disorder. Loss of elastic recoil in the adipose tissue means that fluid can be removed quickly to the lymphatics.

The condition appears to be related to rogue genes which code for elastin.

As you can imagine even the early stages of this chronic condition can impact weight gain negatively even if it never develops into the final and more disfiguring stage.

It may be that lipoedema may be a result of a diet that does not contain enough of the amino acid building blocks for elastin.

The four main amino acids are:

- glycine
- alanine
- valine
- proline

The main source of glycine is in gelatinous products and the skin of animals - think bone broth and pork crackling.

Alanine is a non-essential amino acid and is found in in most animal food sources such as

- egg
- dairy
- meat
- fish

Valine can be found in whole grains, soy, cheese, peanuts, mushrooms and most vegetables.

Proline is found in a wide variety of plant and animal sources so a varied diet should provide an individual's needs.

When elastin recoil is damaged then it is even more important to exercise as this will also help the movement of fluid into the lymphatics.

There is an association of lipoedema with metabolic syndrome. Health professionals suggest losing weight in order to ameliorate the effects of these interconnected conditions. If only it was that simple.

Well, it can be made simpler. There is a nutritional substance known as berberine that has many benefits for people with conditions that predispose them to overweight. There are a number of others which are potential allies (see The Lipoedema Diet by Lynne D M Noble) but berberine has a number of therapeutic benefits.

Berberine is a compound found in many plants. It is yellow and tastes bitter. For this reason, although you can buy it in powder form, it is far more judicious buying it in capsules.

It has a number of benefits and these include:

- an anti-inflammatory effect
- weight loss
- preventing insulin resistance and diabetes

- reducing appetite

but these are only some of the many benefits berberine has.

Some people experience nausea and some stomach upsets. On a personal level, I have never experienced negative side effects although I have slow weight loss and reduced appetite.

The half-life of berberine is quite short so it needs to be taken with every meal. Follow the instructions on the package but generally 500mg three times daily would suffice.

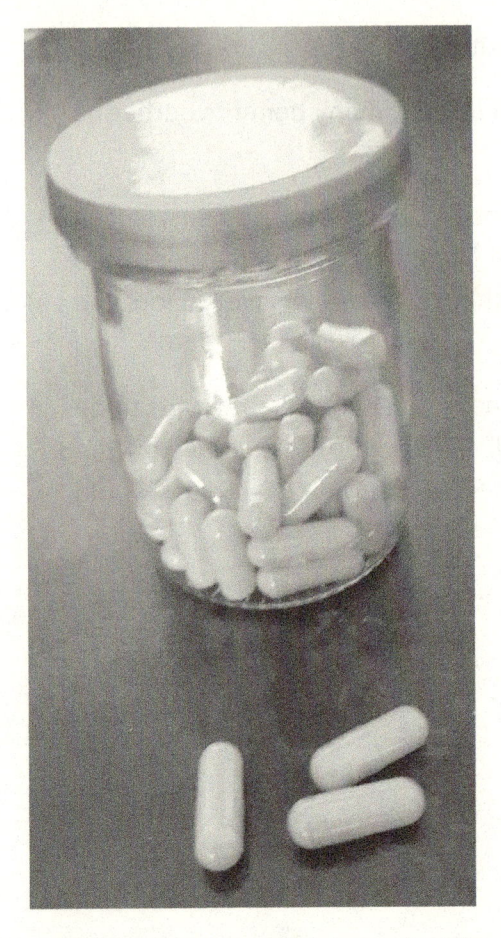

Berberine is an excellent product for those who want to reduce their weight.

Another nutrient that is also useful in the battle against weight gain is that of choline. Choline is a vital nutrient for weight reduction.

Weight reduction is part of the fight in reducing the impact of lipoedema. It is also a hard fight since when we reduce calories and body mass decreases, the synthesis of the hunger inhibiting hormone, leptin, is also reduced. As a result, hunger pangs increase and it is not long before the diet is abandoned without achieving its aims.

How then can we lose weight without damaging muscle mass and further, making sure that this is undertaken without too much effort on our part?

Food is meant to be enjoyed and there is little enjoyment in it when every calorie is being counted on a day to day basis.

A recently discovered nutritional substance which is present in some foods has been found to be the dieter's best friend. Its name is choline and some choline is made in the body but most has to be provided in the food that we eat. Unfortunately, most people are deficient in this vitamin like substance.

What does choline do to help weight loss? Well, choline has been found to help the body use fat as a fuel and further, choline helps to remove excess fat from the blood. When fat is used as a fuel then hunger will not occur.

Studies[3] on the effect of choline supplementation on rapid weight loss and biochemical variables among female taekwondo and judo athletes have born this out. For a number of reasons, it is necessary for athletes to lose weight before important matches. This is undertaken using a number of nutritional substances of which one is choline. Dramatic weight loss without the loss of muscle mass has been observed in those taking choline supplementation.

The athletes took 2g of choline daily divided into two 1g doses for one week. The results indicated a 10.23% change in loss of body fat. The results support the hypothesis that choline could be used to lose weight rapidly without detriment to other body systems.

Good sources of choline are eggs and liver. Two eggs provide about half of the choline requirements for the day.

A Recommended Daily Allowance has not been established for choline since it is a fairly newly discovered substance. However, an Adequate Intake has been established and this is:

- 425mg for women
- 550mg for men

---

[3] https://www.ncbi.nlm.nih.gov/pmc/articles/PMC4096089/#b4-jhk-40-77

Some individuals will require less than this and others more. There are a number of groups of people who are likely to require more and, as such be at risk of being deficient in choline. These groups are:

- Anyone with a poor diet or malabsorption problems
- Pregnant mothers
- Nursing mothers
- The elderly
- Vegetarians and vegans

The best sources of choline are foods which are now advised as those that may increase cholesterol levels. As such they are generally avoided. In addition, the best source of choline – beef liver - has fallen out of popularity. When we take eggs and liver out of the diet then it can be seen that achieving the adequate intake of choline is not easy.

Foods containing choline

- One large egg: 120mg
- Beef liver: one slice contains 280mg
- Salmon: 4 ounces contains 65mg
- Cod: 85gms contains 250mg
- Cauliflower: 120ml contains 25mg
- Broccoli: 120ml contains 24mg
- Brussels sprouts: one cup cooked 65mg
- Soybean oil: one tablespoon contains 47mg

- Peanut butter: one tablespoon 10mg

It can be see that it is considerably harder to obtain adequate intakes of choline in a plant based diet than it is for those who include meat in their meals.

There is no fear in eating eggs. One of choline's functions is to lower cholesterol levels and as eggs contain superb amounts of choline then the hype that they can contribute to heart disease and stroke is unfounded. Choline can also lower blood pressure.

It makes sense to increase levels of choline in the diet. This is not an overly difficult thing to achieve. For example, stirring a couple of egg yolks into mashed potato before topping a shepherd's pie or making proper Crème Anglaise with egg yolks goes well towards the Adequate Intake of choline. Making a shepherd's pie with minced liver is also a tried and tested recipe in our household. I make this with lamb's liver as the flavour is more delicate than that of beef liver. However, it depends on individual taste. Liver is such a good all round food that it is eaten twice weekly in our house.

If cooking is not your forte, then supplements are useful and easily obtainable online and in health food stores. It is recommended that no more than 600mg is taken daily but be guided by the instructions on the pack.

Lymphoedema

Lymphoedema also causes weight gain. Lymphoedema causes swelling. Although most of the swelling tends to be in the arms or legs, it can actually occur anywhere. Lymphoedema may be due to injury that damages the lymph nodes. A blockage forms preventing lymph from draining well.

Ehlers Danlos Syndrome appears to be a risk factor for lymphoedema.

There are a number of treatments for this chronic condition including compression garments, exercise and manual lymphatic drainage. The compression garments are heavy, difficult to put on and extremely warm. Heat and pressure may cause a rebound effect and a worsening of the condition in some people.

More recent studies have found that lymphoedema is due to chronic inflammation. As such there are dietary remedies which can be found in my book The Lymphoedema Diet.

Exercise and the supplement berberine should also be considered as part of the treatment plan for lymphoedema.

More recent studies have highlighted the vital part that two electrolytes play in reducing weight gain and ameliorating the effects of related conditions.

Potassium particularly has not been given the recognition that it deserves. It is time that it was revisited.

The role of potassium in weight loss

While most studies focus on calorie reduction of carbohydrates and fat to reduce the impact of metabolic syndrome, more recent studies[4] have looked at the impact of electrolytes in this process. In particular, increments in dietary potassium has been found to predict weight loss during treatment of metabolic syndrome and obesity.

Potassium has not generally been seen as a major contributor in responding to weight gain. Most people have heard of potassium but there has been little in the media to suggest that there is a deficiency of this mineral cum electrolyte in the population as a whole.

However, potassium is a vital mineral and an electrolyte. It is essential for enabling your muscles to work effectively. This also includes muscles like your heart and the ones that control breathing. Individuals with low potassium levels often have digestive problems like slow bowel transit which may result in constipation and

---

[4]

https://www.ncbi.nlm.nih.gov/pmc/articles/PMC6627830/#:~:text=It%20is%20notable%20that%20the,and%20in%20overall%20caloric%20intake.

impaction. Just walking may be problematical; legs may feel heavy and taking steps an effort. Brain fog and the inability to remember recent events may also be due to low potassium levels.

The importance of potassium in lymphoedema – which often occurs alongside metabolic syndrome – cannot be underplayed either. Unlike the circulatory system, which does have a pump to enable blood to be distributed around the body – the lymphatic system does not. However, the potassium channels are vital to lymph pump activity, formation and its transportation. Without adequate potassium, lymphatic fluid is hampered and may account for the development of secondary lymphoedema.

As lymphoedema and lipoedema often occur alongside each other, then improving potassium intake in cases of deficiency for lipoedema may also help ameliorate this condition.

There have been a number of studies that have shown an association between lymphoedema and some lung problems. When it affects the head and neck this generally occurs at the same time as any external swelling. Changes in voice quality may occur. The voice may be more raspy, singers may not be able to reach the notes that they could do. Difficulty in swallowing or a sense of something stuck in the back of the throat often occurs. This often leads to people swallowing air in an effort to dislodge whatever is stuck in the back of the throat. Breathing may become more laboured.

Diuretics are frowned upon if you have lymphoedema purely because when fluid is lost then lymph becomes thicker and does not flow as easily. The importance of the pumping action required to move lymph has not gained as much publicity. The connection between metabolic syndrome, low potassium levels, abdominal obesity and lymphoedema does not appear to have been given the importance that it deserves in research. There is very little of this nature to be found.

A number of medications can cause low potassium levels. (hypokalaemia) Most notably the non-potassium sparing diuretics like Furosemide while ridding the body of excess fluid also carry with it important minerals like potassium and magnesium. Insulin also causes more potassium to be removed from the blood to cells and can result in a temporary hypokalaemia. Ace inhibitors and non-steroidal anti-inflammatory drugs also have the capacity to raise potassium levels.

There are also potassium sparing diuretics which have the potential to raise potassium levels so you need to ascertain which one you have as this can influence how you approach your dietary intake.

Low potassium levels are associated with low magnesium levels. Magnesium is one of the minerals lost during diuretic use. In addition, many studies show that a greater percentage of the population are deficient in magnesium due to poor diets. The impact of poor nutrition and the side effects of diuretic medication have the ability to cause poor health.

Magnesium is a cofactor in more than 300 enzyme systems. These systems regulate a diversity of biochemical reactions in the body. These include blood glucose control, protein synthesis, blood pressure regulation, among many others. In relation to potassium, it has a role to play in actively transporting calcium and potassium ions across cell membranes. This is necessary for normal heart rhythm, muscle contraction and the conduction of nerve impulses.

The concept of prescribing diuretics to reduce blood pressure is a peculiar one. Low potassium levels will raise your blood pressure as well as giving a propensity to a pot belly. Low potassium levels also encourage the build-up of visceral fat which pumps out inflammatory chemicals.

In the study referred to above, the first 68 participants aged between 18 and 70 years completed a full year's intervention. During this time, they were expected to complete 150 minutes of exercise weekly. In addition, calories were restricted by 25-30% of the normal metabolic resting rate.

The participants were seen by a nutritionist and a physician on a regular basis. The differences were examined after one year.

In that year, participants lost on average 9.36kg. This represented up to a 16.4% reduction in body mass index. Analysis revealed that the percentage change was related to the consumption of potassium, vitamin B6, caporic acid, calcium, sugars and total energy consumption. However, the increase in potassium intake was the strongest indicator of reduction of the BMI closely followed by caproic acid (found in goat's milk).

The range within which potassium works without problems is narrow but any excess is cleared away by the kidneys providing, of course, that the kidneys are functioning correctly.

The Dietary Recommended Intake of potassium is not reached by most people in Western countries. The study showed that the average daily potassium intake in adults was 2.9 - 3.2 for men (DRI is 4.7g. In women this was found to be even less at 2.1-2.3g. Taking this further, the findings were that only 10% of men and only 1% of women were reaching their DRI of potassium.

It has been suggested that low potassium levels are unlikely to be caused by poor dietary habits. The reasoning behind this is that many foods contain potassium including:

- Dark leafy greens
- Potatoes
- Bananas
- Fish
- beans

Bananas particularly are advertised as a good source of potassium and they are but they still only provide one tenth of our daily potassium needs. Potatoes, once found on a daily basis in various forms on our plates have now been replaced with rice, pasta and other grains. Our diets have changed and, as such, the nutrients we ingest have changed. These changes bring new health conditions with them while others will shuffle away.

In addition, when calorie reduction is undertaken, it is highly likely that there is a reduction in the intake of food and food choices. The knock on effect of this is that potassium intake is likely to be reduced as well. Calorie reduction may then not aid weight loss leading to a frustrating and fruitless attempt to lose weight before any thoughts of dietary responses to health conditions are abandoned altogether.

Potassium supplementation is not generally recommended because it is only safe within narrow limits. For this reason, supplements are only found in

99mg doses. Generally, up to 4 daily are recommended but this amount is often less than you would find in one banana. GP's may prescribe higher doses but this generally after tests for suspected potassium deficiency.

Home tests are not available for potassium deficiency.

Some foods which contain reasonable amounts of potassium are:

food	Amount of potassium
Decaffeinated expresso coffee	One cup of prepared coffee 116mg
Low sodium baking powder	560mg
Tomato juice l00mg	229 mg in
Banana l00g	358mg
I cup of strong black tea	90mg
Potato 100g	421 mg
Spinach - one cupful – approx. 30mg	170mg
Milk 240g	366mg
Mushroom 100g	318mg
Cucumber one cup	200mg of potassium
Melon 100g	270mg
Nectarine 100g	200mg
Dates 100mg	656 mg
Dried apricots 100mg	1162mg
Baked beans100mg	358mg

- note: one 1000mg is equal to one g
- one ml is equal to one mg

A useful link for those wishing to increase their potassium intake can be found here.

https://louisville.edu/medicine/departments/familymedicine/files/Potassium%20Food%20List.pdf

However, from the above it should be clear that it is not always that easy to take in the DRI of potassium especially for those who do not have well planned and diverse diets and are restricting calories too.

It is clearly important to remember that without adequate magnesium, potassium – no matter how much you ingested – would simply not be available to the body.

The study found that 37 subjects increase their potassium and 27 decreased this mineral. After one year it was found that those who increased their potassium had a greater weight loss than those who decreased their ingestion of potassium during calorie restriction.

It is always a useful exercise to jot down your food intake over a period of 3 days to ascertain if your diet does contain enough potassium and magnesium.

What is unfair is that any weight gain immediately worsens these two conditions resulting in further development of the symptoms and a further predisposition towards weight gain.

Allergies, Angioedema and Mast Cell Activation Syndrome

Comorbid with connective tissue disorders, including EDS, can be found a predisposition to allergies and angieoedema. The latter is almost always found alongside Mast Cell Activation Disorder. (MCAD).

People with allergies are prone to asthma, eczema, hives and food intolerances.

Asthmatics nearly always are given inhalers which contain steroids in order to control the condition. The problem with steroids is that they cause weight gain. They increase appetite, ramp up your blood sugar levels and reduce your immune system's ability to do its job.

The medical profession will tell you that the effects of inhalers or steroid nasal drops for stuffy noses are not systemic in their effect. They most certainly are.

2015 was a particularly bad year for the appearance of my allergies. Initially I was placed on Nasocort. It worked wonderfully well. I also put on half a stone in a month. I stopped taking the Nasocort and my weight dropped back to what it had been. I tried this regime three more times with the same effect. I stopped taking Nasocort for good.

I was also placed on a steroid inhaler. It did not appear to make much difference apart from the fact that I put on weight but lost it when I stopped using it.

The difficulty with steroids is that it damages connective tissue by thinning it. In people with EDS their connective tissue is already formed improperly.

In the end I did not need an inhaler for my asthma because it was found that I had a five-inch (12cm) gap between my abdominal muscles where the connective tissue between them had torn. This probably describes well how fragile the connective tissue in EDS is.

That was another five inches added to my waist which certainly wasn't fat. It was purely the result of a separating of my abdominal wall.

I underwent a nine-hour operation (Keel repair) to sew everything back into place. I have not had asthma, nor pneumonia, since. It is almost certain that my 'asthma' was caused by gastric fluid travelling back up my oesophagus and into my lungs causing an inflammatory response there.

However, due to prolonged periods of prescribed steroids for repeated bouts of pneumonia - which as it turned out was exacerbated by this abdominal gap, not asthma – my pear shaped figured morphed into the dreaded apple form. This is a known side effect of steroids. The apple shape is frowned upon by medics.

Abdominal obesity, as seen in the apple shape - appears to pump out inflammatory substances with gusto and it is associated with metabolic syndrome.

Metabolic syndrome puts you at greater risk of coronary heart disease and stroke.

This tale does bring us nicely onto the impact of antihistamines on weight.

Antihistamines are purported to have a similar chemical structure as psychotic drugs. Psychotic drugs are well known for causing weight gain. However, the main contributor to weight gain is the impact on histamine by antihistamines.

Histamine is a neurotransmitter. That is, it helps relay messages in the brain and keeps you alert. It is one reason that taking antihistamines makes you tired.

Histamine also relays the 'I'm full' signal. When antihistamines are taken this signal is not activated and it is quite likely that overeating will take place since there is nothing to tell you when to stop.

Thus antihistamines can cause weight gain on a number of levels. Some of the culprits are:

- Certirizine
- Benadryl
- Allegra

- Piriton

But really any antihistamine that causes sleepiness is likely to have the added risk of weight gain. These antihistamines are the ones that are able to breach the blood brain barrier and are antagonistic to histamine.

The weight gain is not minor either. Studies have shown that people on antihistamines tend to be two stone heavier than those who are not taking antihistamines. That is a huge amount.

Further, there is an increased risk of dementia for those taking antihistamines so alternative ways of controlling allergies needs to be seriously considered.

There are gels for smearing inside the nostrils to catch pollen.

High doses of vitamin C are known to control allergies. In addition, it is good for building up collagen, the major protein of connective tissue.

Quercetin also appears to control allergies well with none of the side effects of antihistamines.

There is one antihistamine that does not cross the blood brain barrier and thus does not disrupt satiety signals nor induce drowsiness. This antihistamine is Loratidine and is sold over the counter quite cheaply. Some individuals say that it does not work as well as the ones that pass through the blood brain barrier but if I had to choose an antihistamine- taking everything into consideration - this is the one that I would choose.

Angieoedema

Angieoedema has processes in common with allergies but the swelling tends to be in the deeper layer of tissue rather than manifested superficially.

People with angieoedema may have to use an Epipen if the swelling occurs in the throat area. The swelling often fluctuates but can add a considerable amount of (fluid) weight if not controlled properly,

Mast cells are cells of the immune system that cause allergy like symptoms as soon as the allergen is come into contact with.

Mast cells release substances that are responsible for the symptoms which include swelling and itching.

Really, mast cells can be activated by all manner of substances which include:

- Insect venom
- Infections
- Medications

Many people, as I do, have an idiopathic form of angieoedema. This means that the cause is unknown. This does not mean that there isn't a cause only that no one has yet identified what that cause is.

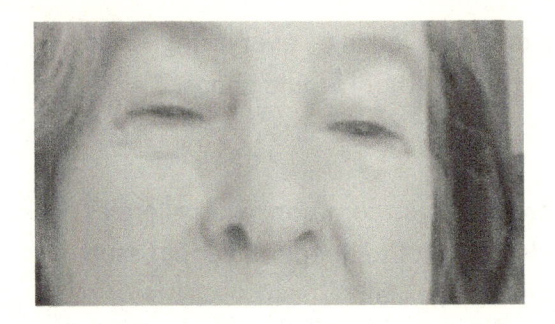

Orbital swelling

There are physical causes and these include heat and pressure. If I wear tight clothing, then my skin swells and itches. It is up to me to make sure that my clothing is loose and cool.

I do have an Epipen because I went through a long phase of throat swelling. I could recognise it as soon as it started because my voice took on a more musical timbre and I began to have swallowing problems.

This went on for three years. No cause was identified but it was recommended by the immunology department in that I have an Epipen, take high doses of Fexofenadine and Tranexamic acid.

The latter two medications made me severely ill and they were abandoned in a short time. I wasn't a fan of antihistamines because of their association with weight gain, anyway. I tried a few different antihistamines to try and find some that I could cope with.

Then a number of changes occurred in my life which reduced the stress that I had been experiencing, quite markedly. I found the angioedema simply melted away during this period. I had heard of this phenomenon happening with angioedema.

Why would this be? During stress a substance called bradykinin is released. Bradykinin is intimately connected with angioedema. It does this by increasing vasodilation and tissue permeability which in turn, results in oedema.

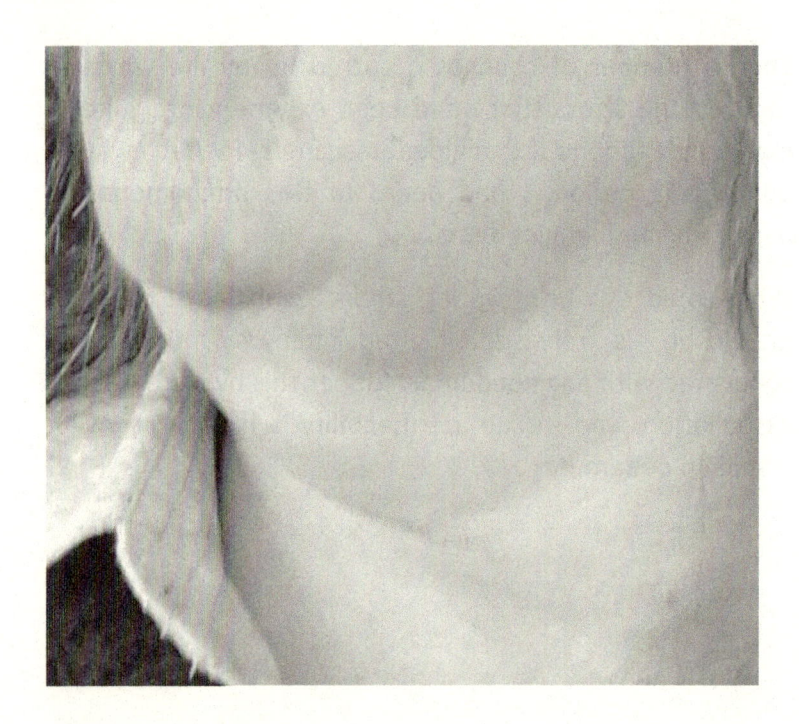

angieoedema of throat

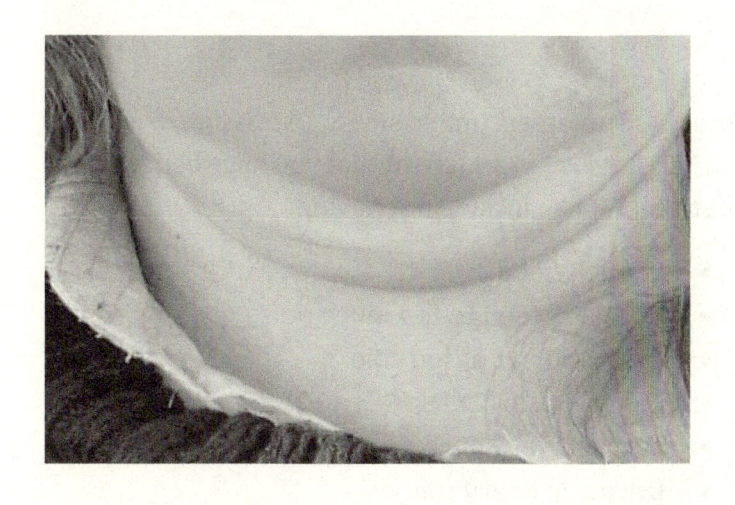

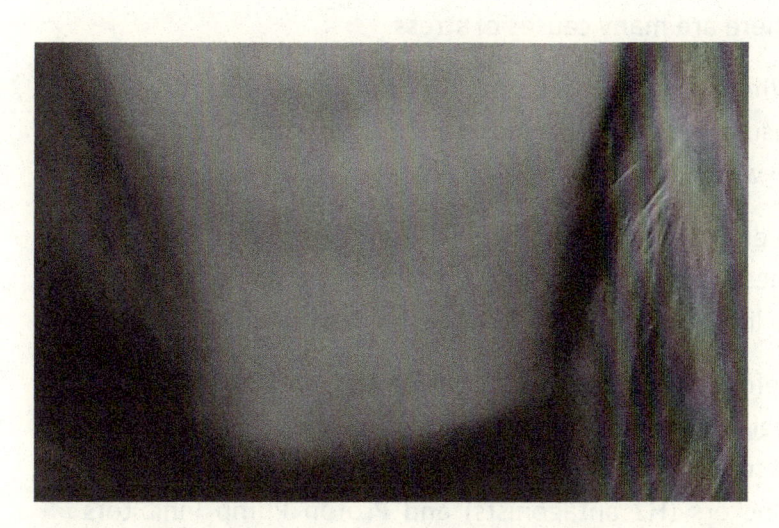

Profile when angioedema isn't present. This photo was taken less than 24 hours after the previous one.

Cortisol is also released under stress. Stressful events abound. It is not just an argument that you have had with your teenager. It can include not having

- Enough sleep
- Being exposed to too much noise
- Being too hot or too cold
- Being in pain
- Taking an exam
- Driving in heavy traffic
- Not having enough money to live on

There are many causes of stress.

When cortisol levels rise, we can be insulin resistant. Insulin resistance increases blood sugar and predisposes to weight gain and potentially Type 2 diabetes.

Even if an individual lived without exposure to many of these stressors, the fact is that EDS is a major challenge to live with and therefore has its own inbuilt stressors.

Before we leave this subject of medications that cause weight gain through a variety of mechanisms, we ought of examine another group of medications called H2 blockers (H2 antagonists) and Proton Pump Inhibitors (PPI's) that are routinely used for conditions such as gastric ulcers and gastroesophageal reflux disorder which is often shortened to GERD.

GERD is a very common problem in those with EDS due to lax tissues. H2 blockers and PPI's such as Lansoprazole did not directly alter appetite but they do contribute to obesity indirectly.

A study[5] of the relationship between these medications and weight gain concluded

PPI use was associated with a significant weight gain in men and a non-significant weight gain in women. Measures of energy intake physical activity and sedentary behaviour were similar between PPI users and non-users in both men and women.

Before we look at another (non-medication) cause for gaining weight. It would be useful to look at some other medications that are routinely prescribed, all of which have well documented side effects of gaining weight through oedema.

These include:
- Non-steroidal anti-inflammatory drugs
- Drugs for high blood pressure
- Oestrogens
- Thiazolidinedione (diabetic medicine)

---

[5] https://www.ncbi.nlm.nih.gov/pmc/articles/PMC4632436/

- Psychoactive medications such as antidepressants, some antipsychotics and lithium

Many people with EDS are on numerous medications to help them cope with the symptoms of having this condition.

To put things into perspective, if an individual takes antihistamines. NSAID's and anti-depressants, then we are looking at a potential weight gain of three to four stone which is not related to over-eating.

Many people with EDS are on far more medications than this.

Fortunately, one of the building blocks of collagen is a non-essential amino acid called glycine. It is an inhibitory neurotransmitter and slows down pain signals. Therefore, it is an effective pain reliever without the side effects that come with NSAID's. In addition, it also helps sleep.

Glycine can be obtained online and at most health food stores as a supplement but really the best source is bone broth and gelatinous products.

If you do use a supplement. then it comes as in granular form. It is slightly sweet and can be added to cereals and yogurt, cake mixes or into drinks.

Thiazolidinedione (diabetic medicine) could be replaced with berberine that encourages weight loss. Studies have shown berberine to be as effective as Metformin.

I am always concerned that individuals who have a condition that is related to weight are then prescribed medication to control the condition but, in the process it causes weight gain.

It doesn't make sense really,

However, please remember that any changes in medication should be discussed with your health professional before going ahead,

In addition, some chronic conditions which may be insidious in nature may go undetected for months or even years before symptoms become too obvious to ignore. These conditions also cause weight gain. They include

- Congestive heart failure
- Kidney disease

But this is by no means a definitive list. This is why when unexpected weight changes occur they should not be assumed to have no cause but that of taking in too many calories.

A verbalised belief like this only hinders the patient/health professional relationship.

At the very least, there should be a medication review against a list of medications known to cause weight gain.

The thyroid needs to be checked to see if it is functioning normally.

How the condition impacts the ability to exercise and shop and prepare food also needs to be considered. EDS can make it difficult if not impossible to buy and prepare the bespoke diet that EDSer's need.

The belief that weight gain is entirely due to more calories going in than expended is erroneous and judgemental. Weight gain has a number of diverse causes and it needs to be investigated sympathetically and without judgement.

All health professionals need to learn to really listen and not discount any of the patient's verbalised experiences or thoughts on the subject. They may sound implausible at the time but they may just hold the key to why certain symptoms have manifested themselves.

Even if it is eventually established that a patient is contributing to weight gain by their eating patterns, there is still a reason why this occurs and this reason needs to be established and addressed. Some of these reasons may include:

- Boredom
- Anxiety (carbohydrates help alleviate anxiety)
- Pain
- Lack of knowledge about healthy eating
- Financial restrictions

Again this is not a definitive list. The more a health professional gently explores, the more they learn.

One of my patients had had a very traumatic life, often going without food to feed her children. Eventually, her life improved but she still felt obliged to eat anything before her in case the next meal did not come along. Difficult circumstances may leave us but that does not mean that we automatically leave the behaviours behind that have helped us survive those difficult times.

Survival behaviour is the hardest to change.

However, just to underline that oedema is a major contributory cause to weight gain in EDS. It does need to be dealt with as some of the ongoing complications may become permanent.

This list of symptoms may help in identifying it.

Untreated oedema may cause

- Stretched skin – this may become itchy and resemble urticaria (hives).
- Painful swelling. You may recognise this as when you touch that part of your body against something, it is painful.
- Stiffness in joints.
- Increase risk of infection in the area.
- Difficulty in walking. If this occurs in the abdominal area, then it can actually throw you off balance.
- Due to the fluid build-up there is also an increased chance of infection. Scarring may occur between layers of tissue increasing the risk of pain and infection even further.

- Loss of sensation in the swollen area.
- The blood vessels may lose their elasticity even more than EDS already does causing a further build-up of fluid.
- Poor blood circulation

This is why it is so important to recognise and deal with oedema as soon as possible.

Many years ago I complained to my GP that I could not stand against the sink to wash up because pressing up against it felt so tender.

Instead of investigating further, it was left because it did not appear to be something that was within my GP's experience. The knock on effect of this was that I continued to be in pain for far too long. I did not feel that I could trust my GP and eventually moved.

My new GP's were just lovely. They did not immediately have all the answers. Sometimes they would just say, 'Lynne you are a conundrum,' but they never poured scorn on what I said. They acknowledged that they did not have all the answers but were prepared to look for them.

Eventually, I was referred to rheumatology where they were able to put all the diverse amount of symptoms together as manifestations of EDS.

This was a culmination of a quest for me. I had noticed early on in my life that many family members suffered a variety of apparently unrelated symptoms and inexplicable pain. I made it my work to give this elusive phenomenon a name.

I was in my fifties before I had the answers that I needed.

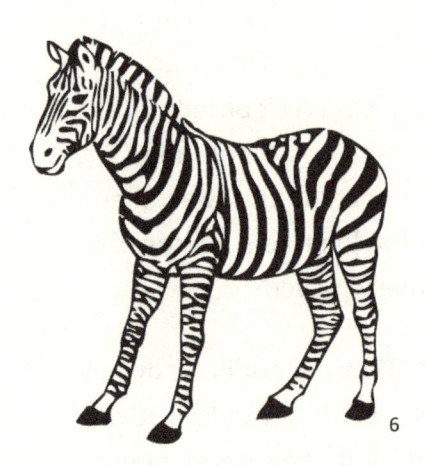

---

[6] http://clipart-library.com/free/zebra-black-and-white-clipart.html

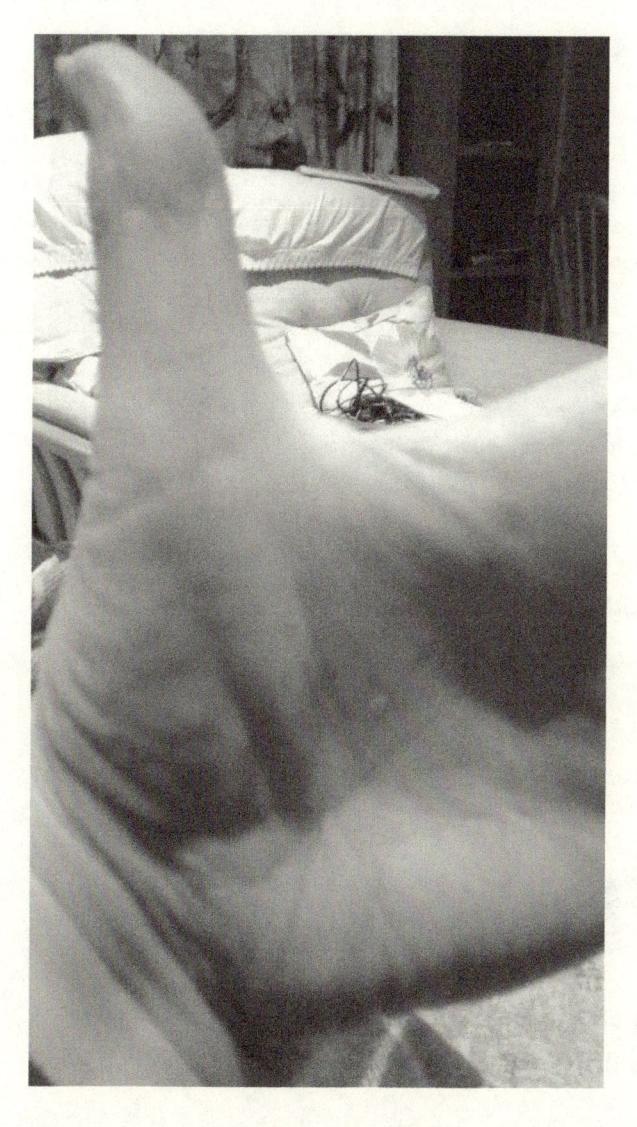

Note the swelling of the tissues below the author's hand

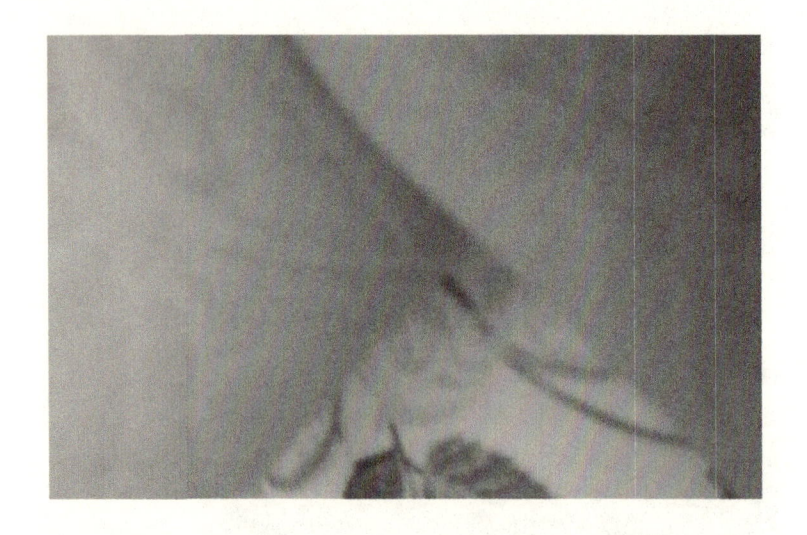

Angieoedema causes marked dermographics. This skin writing is another sign of fluid retention.

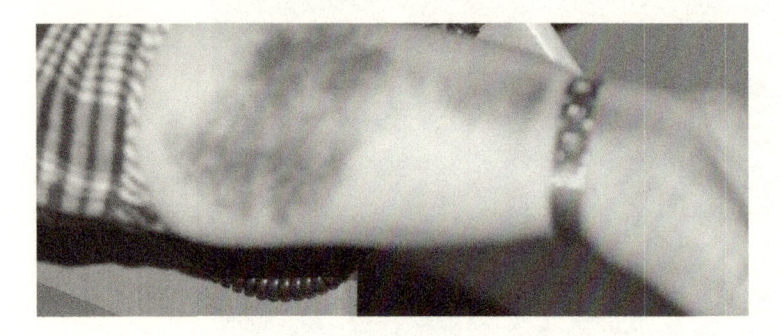

People with EDS tend to bruise easily. When damage to tissue occurs there will also be oedema.

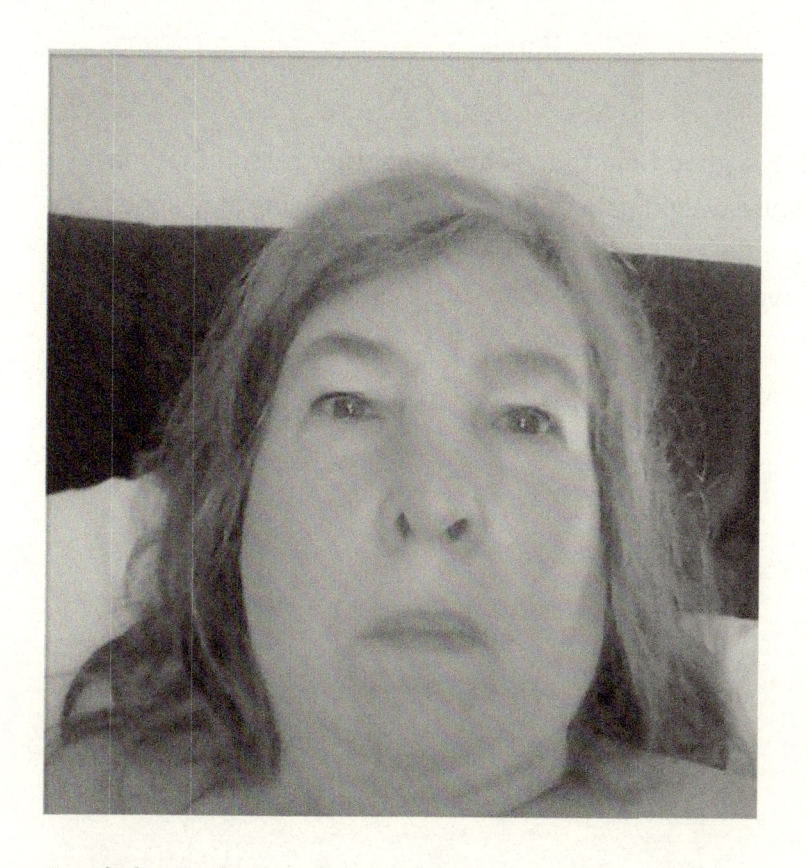

Anaphylactic shock: note increased sweating, swelling in throat area as well as face. The nostril is distorted due to the build-up of fluid.

It is a good time to look at yet another reason that may cause weight gain. At first what I am saying may appear a little contradictory but stick with it and all will be revealed.

Long Term Protein Deficiency

Protein is a macronutrient. A macronutrient is a substance that is required in large amounts for the health of the human body.

There are a diverse number of types of protein in the human body. You will be familiar with some of these. EDSer's will have heard of collagen which is the major protein found in connective tissue. Another well-known protein is keratin. Hair and nails are made of this protein.

Proteins are made of building blocks called amino acids. A different mix of amino acids will produce a different protein with different characteristics.

An analogy is that if you have twenty ingredients in your cupboard and you mix a few out of the total together and then do the same but add one or two different ingredients then your final result may well look very different.

Take this recipe

Flour + butter + sugar + eggs = cake mix

Take the eggs out and you will make a crumble mix. They have different properties and are used for different purposes.

You can see that if you don't have the full complement of ingredients (amino acids) in the right amounts then your final composition will not be up to the job it was intended to do.

Protein makes up about 18% of a person's body weight. You cannot build muscle, skin, hair, joints bones, organs etcetera, without protein.

Proteins are needed to make enzymes.

Enzymes are generally made from protein. They are biological molecules that speed up the rate of the chemical reactions that occur in your cells.

Without them proper digestion of a meal might take days or weeks. They are required for metabolic processes. Metabolic processes change food into energy which is vital to sustain all parts of life.

Without enzymes we cannot function. We cannot think, move, grow, and so on, without optimal metabolic processes. This also includes maintaining homeostasis.

Homeostasis is the balancing act which occurs between interdependent processes going on in the body. When homeostasis is not in harmony then oedema frequently occurs.

Due to the complexity of EDS and its widely diverse symptoms, appetite may not always be maintained. People with gastroparesis may not want to eat as they feel that it will add further to the discomfort that they feel, for example. This is understandable. However, severe long term protein deficiency can cause oedema as well as worsen existing symptoms. After all, you require enzymes not only to help digest food but to help build and maintain the gastrointestinal lining and remove fluid in and out of cells as required.

This is why people who have extra nutritional needs are often prescribed protein shakes to be taken in addition to their usual diet.

In its more severe form protein deficiency is known as kwashiorkor. This is a condition caused by inadequate protein intake.

Initial and later symptoms include:

- Lethargy and fatigue
- Irritability
- Loss of muscle mass
- Oedema
- Increased risk of infection
- A swollen belly

Strangely enough it is generally only the latter symptoms that appears to worry people. They react to this by going on a diet thus generally reducing their protein intake even further.

Do not think that Kwashiorkor is only relevant to undeveloped countries.

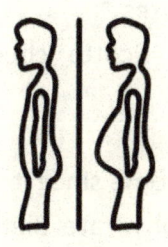

kwashiorkor

[7]

Adequate protein in the diet is one reason why diets such as the high protein Dukan diet is so effective.

The Atkins diet also promotes a high protein/high fat diet.

Slimming World also follow similar lines.

Phase one of the South Beach diet recommend that these foods be eaten

- Lean meat
- Skinless chicken and turkey breast
- Fish and shellfish
- Turkey, bacon and pepperoni

---

[7] dreamstime.com

- Eggs and egg whites
- Soy based meat substitutes
- Low fat hard cheese, ricotta cheese and cottage cheese

The latter may be a good diet for some since it is clearly a very high protein low fat/carbohydrate diet but for people with EDS the chicken skin contains lots of amino acids that help build up collagen. It is nutritious and tasty and should be eaten not thrown away.

I can see why the skin has been removed from the South Beach diet as chicken skin contains a lot of fat but fat in itself will not promote weight gain otherwise the Atkins diet would not be so effective.

To lay down fat you need to increase insulin levels. Protein and fat hardly make a mark on insulin levels. It is the simple carbohydrates that do this such as:

- Products made with white flour
- Sugar
- White rice

Simple carbohydrates also attract fluid into the cells thus promoting mild fluid retention.

Of course inadequate protein intake also produces poor muscle mass and poor muscle mass also means that fewer calories are burned.

The dreaded bingo wings are not generally due to overweight but to loss of muscle. It is a common process in ageing and is known as sarcopenia.

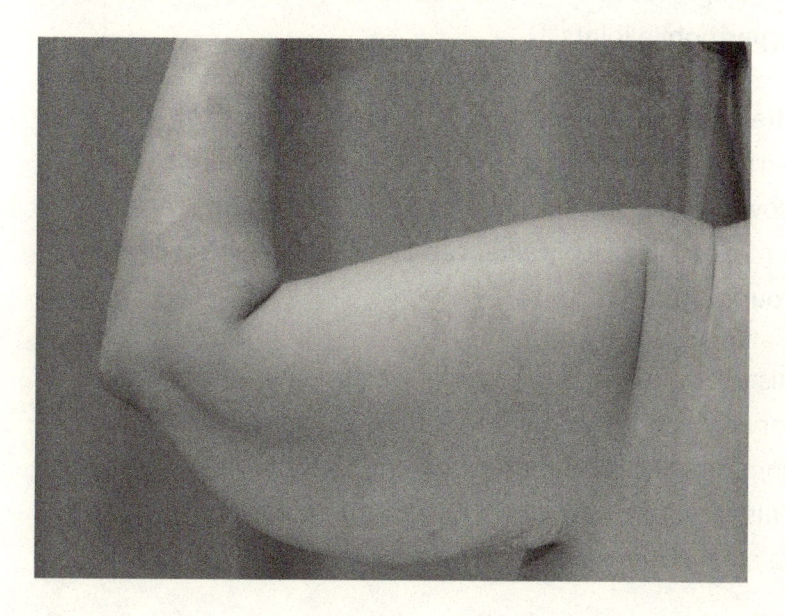

8

There is such a condition known as sarcopenia obesity. The impact of sarcopenia obesity and its impact for

---

[8] http://georgemustloseweight.blogspot.com/2009/05/bingo-wings.html

weight gain and loss of toning in the body should not be underestimated. Due to pain and the risk of subluxations and dislocations. For example, in those with EDS, the building up of muscle mass is important. Working alongside a knowledgeable and sympathetic physiotherapist is of paramount importance especially as building muscle mass helps to stabilise those hypermobile joints.

There are a number of simple exercises such as lifting fairly light weights which can help build muscle mass slowly. You don't need expensive equipment. A four-pint plastic milk container can be adapted quite easily for your purpose.

Just fill it to a comfortable weight and extend arms forward and then to the side. Once you can move comfortably, increase the water in the container slightly. This may take a couple of weeks but every fortnight, aim to add another 100ml to the weight.

You will know when you have built muscle mass because the task while initially hard will become too easy. It is at this point you can increase the weight of the container by adding a little more water.

Figure 1. Body Composition Changes with Sarcopenic Obesity. As people age they lose the lean muscle mass gained in young adulthood (A), resulting in a higher proportion of fat mass (B), even if the absolute amounts of body fat remain constant. This can lead to sarcopenic obesity—a loss of muscle and a concomitant increase in fat, often while body weight remains stable or even decreases. Illustration by Anne Rains.

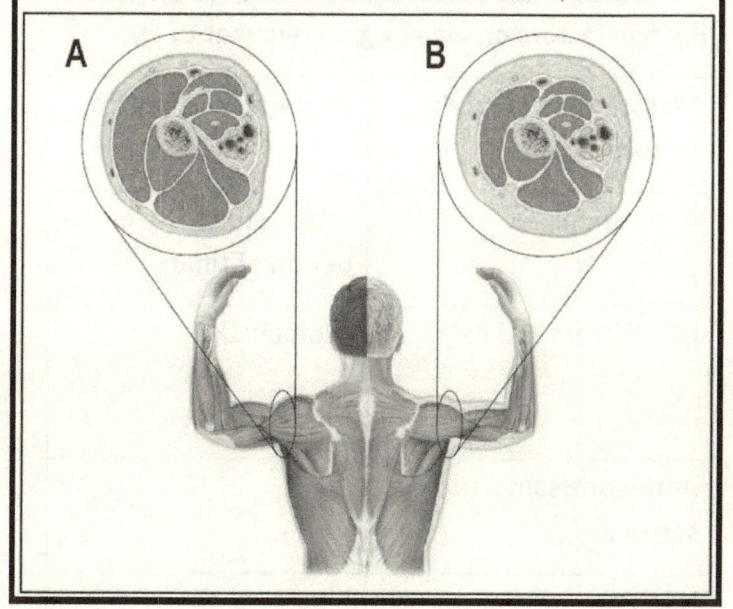

---

[9] Fanatic cook.com

I think it is important at this stage in the book that the impact of various medications and other phenomenon that contribute to weight gain - that are particularly relevant to those with EDS - are tabulated. Here goes.

Table showing the impact of medications and lifestyle factors on weight gain relevant to EDS.

Medications/lifestyle factors	Average weight gain
Antihistamines	Two stone over a period of time
H2 blockers and PPI	Women 1kg Men 2 kg
Antidepressants such as sertraline	10lb
NSAID's	5lb
Steroids such as prednisolone	5lb
Antidiabetics like thiazolidinedione	10lb
Beta blockers	Up to 3lb

High carbohydrate diet	Up to 5lb just in fluid retention
High salt diet	Up to 3lb in water retention
Inadequate protein diet	7lb in fluid retention
Anti-psychotics such as risperidone	10lb
Medication for treating anxiety and neuropathic pain like pregabalin and gabapentin	10lb
Venous insufficiency and pedal oedema	3lb

When you consider the above, bearing in mind that many EDSers will be on a number of medications then a non- dietary reason for weight gain and inability to lose weight when on a calorie reducing diet, now becomes clear.

Medications/lifestyle factors	Mechanisms of weight gain
Antihistamines	• Calories cannot be burned effectively when on antihistamines (lower metabolism) • Lack of satiety signal as histamine is blocked so more likely to over eat • The drowsy effects of antihistamines mean that people are less likely to exercise • Higher insulin concentration • Changes in gut microbiome

	cause depressed energy expenditure
H2 blockers and PPI	• Side effect of insomnia is related to weight gain • Constipation • Urinary retention • Allergic reactions
Antidepressants such as sertraline	• Fluid retention • Metabolic changes • Increased appetite due to improved mood
NSAID's	• Fluid retention
Steroids such as prednisolone	• Salt and water retention • Increased appetite

Antidiabetics like thiazolidinedione	• Increase in subcutaneous fat • Fluid retention
Beta blockers	• Metabolic changes • Fluid retention especially if diuretics have been swapped for beta blockers
High carbohydrate diet	• Every gram of glycogen stored in the body attracts 2-3gm's of water.
High salt diet	• Sodium attracts water
Inadequate protein diet	• Osmotic imbalance in the gastrointestinal area leading to

	fluid retention in abdominal area
Anti-psychotics such as risperidone	• Metabolic changes • Fluid retention
Medication for treating anxiety and neuropathic pain like pregabalin and gabapentin	• Affects calcium channels causing swelling • Appetite change • Fatigue – less likely to exercise • Interaction with metabolism • Fluid retention
Venous insufficiency and pedal oedema	Fluid retention

When you consider the above, bearing in mind that many EDSers will be on a number of medications then a non- dietary reason for weight gain and inability to lose weight when on a calorie reducing diet, now becomes clear.

Two Dietary Changes to Consider

I'm not in favour of counting calories. I can see that some individuals like this structured approach and it may work for them. However, it is not realistic given that not all calories are equal, regardless of what the health profession may say.

If you take 100g of protein and 100g of simple carbohydrate the latter will raise insulin levels which will help store fat. The former does not and therefore does not contribute to fat storage. This is the principle behind the Atkins diet. This is a little too simplistic, however, some amino acids which form protein can cause obesity without adequate carbohydrate to provide serotonin. This will be looked at in the chapter, brown fat, white fat, later.

Further, if you reduce calorie intake too much then there is a chance that you will not supply your body with all the nutrients that it needs.

There are really only two dietary changes that I would ask you to consider and neither of them involve a lot of thought.

Inflammation can cause oedema. Some foods are notorious for creating inflammation and the main culprit is a poly unsaturated fatty acid omega 6.

Omega 6 PUFA's can be highly inflammatory in nature as they can produce arachidonic acid. Some inflammation is required for healing damaged tissues but often inflammation becomes out of control and it is then that it causes problems.

PUFA's and arachidonic acid deserve more attention when looking at food substances which may help to progress lipoedema, lymphoedema and generalised fluid retention.

Arichidonic acid is a polyunsaturated omega-6 fatty acid. It is found in the membranes of the body's cells and is particularly abundant in the brain, muscles and liver. It is a key inflammatory intermediate and can act as a vasodilator. This means it can widen blood vessels.

Arichidonic acid has many beneficial roles in the body. It will not cause inflammation unless tiny particles, called electrons, try and disrupt the stability of other electrons found in the fat that forms part of the cell membranes. Eating plenty of antioxidants would prevent this from happening but our current diets are wanting in that:

- We are eating more and more of the omega 6 polyunsaturated fatty acids in our diets than ever before
- Our diets lack enough of the foods which have antioxidant capacity such as fresh fruit and vegetables

Arachidonic acid can be metabolised to both anti-inflammatory and proinflammatory eicanosoids. It is quite likely that if you suffer from joint pain, bronchoconstriction, microvascular permeability or lymphoedema that arachidonic acid has been converted to a pro-inflammatory compound in your body.

> Eicanosoids are a class of compounds (like leukotrienes and prostaglandins) which are synthesised from poly unsaturated fatty acids (PUFA's) - like arachidonic acid – and that are involved in cellular activity. They are lipid mediators of inflammation.

in fact, a study[10] on lymphoedema in breast cancer patients has supported the connection between raised omega 6 PUFA's and lymphoedema.

The study demonstrated that breast cancer survivors with lymphoedema had elevated PUFA's, arachidonic acid, fatty acid desaturase enzyme activity indices and EPA in serum phospholipids.

The study concluded that the extent of fatty acid composition might be related to the risk of secondary lymphoedema in breast cancer survivors.

Where are PUFA's found?

Sources of PUFA's are Canola oil, grapeseed oil, corn oil, soybean oil, peanut oil among others.

There are plenty of hidden sources – granola, crisps, energy bars, flax seeds and commercially raised poultry, beef and eggs all contain PUFA's.

In fact, our consumption of PUFA's has risen dramatically since their introduction into our diets. They have now replaced the more stable saturated fats such as lard, dripping and butter that were the mainstay of the UK diet until around the early 1970's when the apparently 'healthy' benefits of

---

[10] https://www.ncbi.nlm.nih.gov/pubmed/27041742

polyunsaturated fatty acids were heavily marketed and included in many ready meals and snacks.

I know some of you will be convinced that omega 6 oils are healthier than fats like lard and butter but the latter two do not initiate inflammatory processes. Their bonds are saturated and therefore they are not reactive.

Lard doesn't smoke at high temperatures it doesn't break down and pump out harmful free radicals.

Lard has a great deal of monounsaturated fatty acid in its composition. It is rich in oleic acid. This is the same fatty acid as is found in the healthy olive oil.

Really, a return to using lard, butter and dripping in our cooking and diets is far healthier and may reduce many of the oedematous swellings which occur with inflammation.

Nearly all prepacked and ready meals contain omega 6 PUFA's so they are hard to avoid. If you enjoy cooking, then it will not be a problem. Meals are much tastier when butter, lard and dripping are used in their preparation.

The second change that needs to be considered is reducing the amount of simple carbohydrates in your diet. This does not necessarily mean that I would like you to eat fewer calories as that can be counterproductive. However, the simple carbohydrates need to be replaced as much as possible with more sources of protein and the good saturated fats that I have just discussed.

This change will prevent spikes of insulin that are needed to store fat.

In addition, the amount of protein that you eat also determines your food intake. You will continue to feel hungry until you have ingested the amount of protein that your body needs for its growth and maintenance.

If you eat breakfast, then it makes sense to eat a high protein breakfast rather than toast and jam.

Some good quality high protein breakfasts are:

- Bacon, eggs and mushrooms
- Ham omelette
- Selection of cheeses and oatcakes with butter
- Sugar free plain yogurt. Most fruits do raise blood sugar levels very quickly.
- A platter of meat
- A cheeseburger wrapped in a lettuce leaf

The amount of protein foods that you eat are not restricted so if you would like a 4 egg omelette then that is acceptable.

I am sure that you will have your own ideas but basically, the more protein you have earlier in the day, the less likely that you will feel hungry as the day goes on and the less likely you will want to graze as the day goes on.

We seem to have lost all reason as often the biggest meal is late at night which does not prevent the nibbling throughout the day that often leads to weight gain.

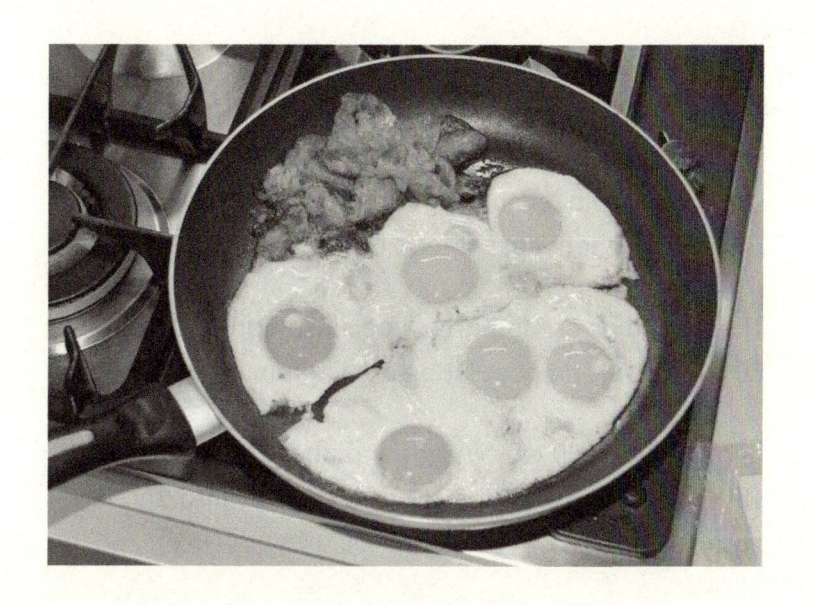

Eggs and bacon, a great high protein breakfast.

Now we have looked at many causes of weight gain that have particular relevance to those with EDS. We have looked at two nutritional substances – berberine and choline – that can help with weight loss. However, there is yet another nutritional substance where a deficiency is implicated in weight gain.

We shall now turn to the subject of vitamin D.

Vitamin D deficiency and weight gain

The role of vitamin D in human health has become studied more in recent years in relation to the inverse relationship between vitamin D levels and obesity.

These studies are important because approximately 80% of the world population are vitamin D deficient.

In one study 400 overweight and obese participants, with vitamin D deficiency were divided into three groups.

The first group did not receive vitamin D supplementation.

The second and third group received 25,000 and 100,000 IU's, monthly, respectively.

After 6 months it was found that the groups that had supplemented with vitamin D had lost weight and had smaller waists.

There are a number of reasons why this may have occurred.

In obesity, vitamin D increases insulin sensitivity and insulin sensitivity is associated with weight loss.

As vitamin D also affects the storage and production of fats, increasing vitamin D to restore levels back to optimum helps to decrease the body fat percentage.

Vitamin D also helps to address systemic inflammation.

Systemic inflammation is often associated with those who are obese with an apple shaped profile.

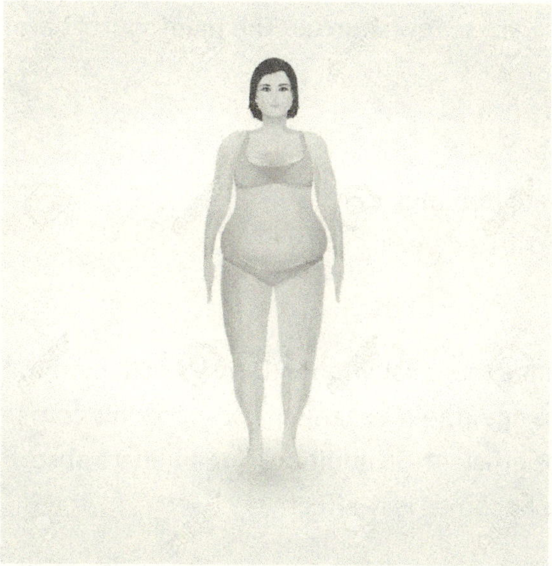

Typical apple shape [11]

---

[11] https://www.123rf.com/photo_53224488_stock-vector-apple-body-shape.html

Vitamin D activates receptors in the pancreatic beta cells. The main function of a beta cell is to produce and secrete insulin.

Insulin helps to regulate levels of glucose in the blood.

Vitamin D is practically impossible to get enough of in diet. There are so few sources. The main sources are:

- Oily fish
- Eggs
- Irradiated mushrooms
- Fortified cereals
- Lard

The sun provides the most vitamin D by its action on the skin but as we age, the mechanism by which this comes about is not as efficient. In addition, our ability to absorb nutrients also becomes less effective.

A number of groups of people are at particular risk of vitamin D deficiency. These include:

- The elderly (those over the age of 55 years)
- People of colour

- People with malabsorption problems such as those with Crohn's disease
- People who remain mainly indoors
- Those on low fat diets as vitamin D needs to be taken with a little fat in order for it to be absorbed.
- Those on a poor diet generally
- Obese people

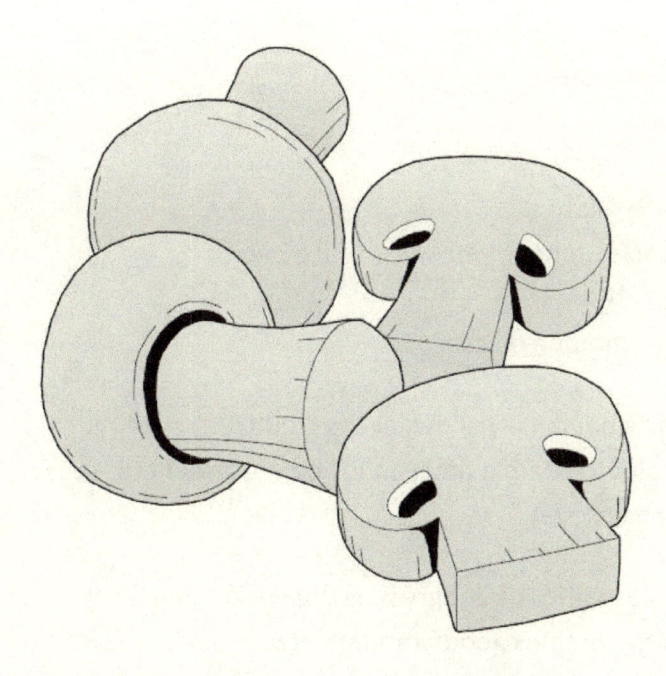

Irradiated mushrooms are a good source of vitamin D

Obese people are at risk because fat cells act as a storage reservoir for vitamin D. The more obese an individual is the greater the storage capacity when really we need vitamin D to be circulating in the body.

The signs of vitamin D deficiency include:

- Hair loss
- Osteopenia
- Osteoporosis
- Frequent infections
- Weight gain
- Fatigue
- Bone pain
- Depression
- Muscle cramps, weakness and aches
- Diabetes
- Autoimmune disease

The recommended daily allowance is 2,000 IU's. Vitamin D is a fat soluble vitamin and cannot be absorbed unless taken with a little fat.

One of the casualties of 'progress' is the discontinued use of lard which contains good amounts of vitamin D.

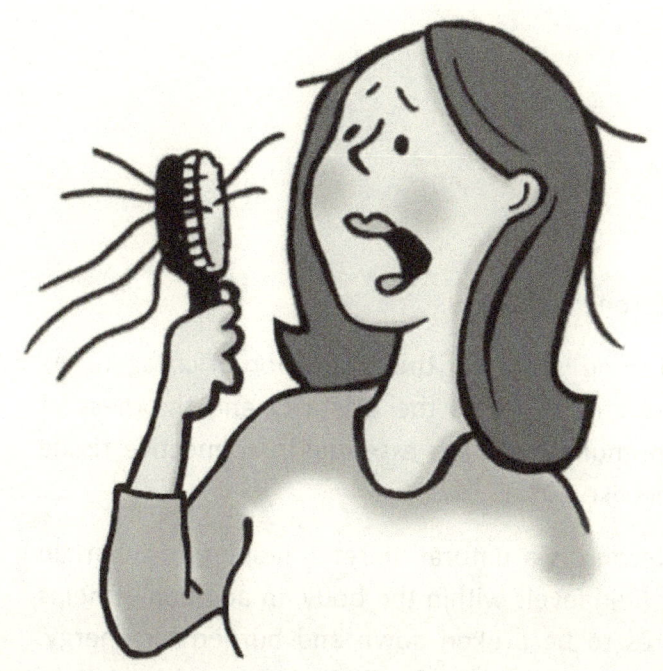

[12] **hair loss is common with vitamin D deficiency**

---

[12] http://clipart-library.com/clipart/279168.htm

85

Progesterone deficiency

Progesterone is vital for the production of collagen. As progesterone increases the elasticity and thickness of skin, optimum levels are essential in connective tissue disorders like EDS.

Progesterone is a natural diuretic, helping to maintain normal fluid levels within the body. In addition, it helps fat stores to be broken down and burned for energy. However, if progesterone levels are low then blood sugar levels rise and muscle tissue is broken down. Cellulite is chronic subcutaneous fat which is often tethered to underlying muscle by connective tissue. This gives it the dimpled appearance.

There are many causes of low progesterone. This condition is not just related to the ageing process. Excess weight will tip the balance in favour of oestrogen dominance. Further, stress will transform progesterone, through action by the kidneys to the stress hormone cortisol.

Cortisol stimulates the metabolism of carbohydrate and fat so that there is a ready supply of energy for the fight or flight response. However, it also stimulates the release of insulin. Insulin is known to increase appetite especially for sweet foods.

Surprisingly, low cholesterol may also contribute hypo-progesterone. The precursor to progesterone is another hormone called pregnenolone. Cholesterol is required for the synthesis of pregnenolone and other hormones. When cholesterol levels are inadequate, then vital hormones cannot be synthesised. In some cases, the synthesis of hormones may be impacted by statins.

Although there are a number of creams which can be rubbed into the skin and are said to raise progesterone levels, many of these contain a substance known as diosgenin. Diosgenin is extracted from the wild yam. However, the human body cannot make progesterone from diosgenin only pregnenolone.

Diet can affect the production of progesterone. Magnesium and vitamin B6 both boost progesterone levels. Indeed, research has shown that high vitamin B6 levels reduce the chance of miscarriage by 50% as well as increasing fertility by 120%. Optimum levels of progesterone are required for the continuation of the pregnancy.

Vitamin B6 is an essential co-factor required for the normal speed of the cross linking of collagen by enzymes. The strength of collagen is partially dependent on this vitamin. When collagen is strengthened then fluid retention is unlikely to occur. Normal elastic recoil enables lymph to drain, too.

The importance of making sure that you have adequate magnesium levels needs to be underlined. Most people are magnesium deficient especially if they are taking diuretics such as Furosemide. As magnesium helps maintain proper fluid balance, taking diuretics can be counterproductive on many counts.

Magnesium is required for the synthesis of collagen and elastin as well as the breakdown of worn out collagen and elastin.

In younger women, optimum levels of zinc increase the level of follicle stimulating hormone (FSH). Once FSH reaches optimum levels ovulation will occur. After ovulation has occurred the ovaries will make progesterone to prepare the uterus for a potential pregnancy.

Vitamin C is the king of vitamins when it comes to raising progesterone levels. Studies have shown that high levels had a significant impact on progesterone levels, increasing the amount by 77% when 750mg were taken daily.

When you consider that the daily recommended amount of vitamin C is 60 mg you can see that this amount is hopelessly inadequate. In fact, this amount was recommended as a sufficient daily intake as it prevented the deficiency disease scurvy. However, although it may prevent scurvy it does not promote optimum health. It is the very minimum that you can get away with in order to maintain life.

Beta carotene is also able to stimulate production of progesterone. Beta carotene is the precursor to vitamin A. Many orange coloured vegetables such as carrots and pumpkin contain good amounts of beta carotene.

Further, vitamin E is able to stimulate production. 150 IU's has been mooted as providing the best benefits. Intakes higher than this may actually be counterproductive. Vitamin E is found in nuts and wheat germ, mainly.

It can be seen that inadequate levels of essential vitamins, macro and trace minerals may contribute to low progesterone levels thus increasing the potential for weight gain and/or fluid retention.

Table of progesterone boosting nutrients, their food sources and mode of action.

Nutrients	Food sources	Mode of action
cholesterol	organ meats, eggs and shellfish. However, the body will naturally make what is required. Statins may interfere with this process.	Cholesterol is required for the synthesis of pregnenolone which is the 'mother' of progesterone.
magnesium	Green leafy vegetables, nuts, dark chocolate, wholegrain bread, meat and dairy	Magnesium boosts the synthesis of progesterone through a series of actions beginning with the regulation of the pituitary gland
Vitamin C	Fresh fruit and vegetables	750mg daily boosts progesterone production by 77%
Vitamin B6	Eggs, pork, poultry, wholemeal grains	• Strengthens collagen cross links. • Enables liver to break

		down oestrogen • Helps stimulate corpus luteum and thus the production of progesterone
Vitamin E	Nut oils and wheat germ	Increases corpus luteum blood flow
Beta carotene	Carrots and pumpkins and other yellow/orange vegetables	Increase in luteal blood flow and size
Zinc	Animal protein, beans and whole wheat products.	Increases the production of FSH which stimulates ovulation and, in turn the production of progesterone

Inflammation

Just what is inflammation? That's probably a good question for many people. We have an idea when we see redness and swelling that inflammation is going on which will always be accompanied by pain. This pain can be diffuse especially when the source is inflammation occurring internally. The pain may also be referred pain so that it appears elsewhere than the original area of injury.

Researchers at the Medical College of Georgia discovered a nerve centre in a cell layer in the spleen that controls the immune response and therefore inflammation throughout the body. It is quelled by taking 2g of baking soda in water for two weeks.

The only downside to this is that this has the potential to raise your blood pressure. If you do have raised blood pressure hen taking 250mg of magnesium and a glass of tomato juice for the potassium will most likely address this.

Trace Elements and Weight

Zinc

Zinc is a trace element which is often associated with the health of the immune system. Indeed, a zinc deficiency is generally associated with vulnerability to infection. Zinc is better known for its ability to activate T lymphocytes. It also has a regulatory role in controlling the immune response as well as attacking cancerous and infected cell. Zinc supplementation studies in the elderly have shown a reduction in the rate and severity of infections, decreased oxidative stress and the presence of fewer inflammatory cytokines. However, its super status is not just confined to the health of the immune system.

Zinc is required for many functions in the body especially in relation to activating enzymes which speed up metabolic processes in the body. Some of these processes may be related to wound healing and age-related chronic diseases such as age-related macular degeneration. However, there are some quite remarkable effects on weight loss when a zinc deficiency is corrected. Zinc has an important role to play in controlling metabolism. Those with a zinc deficiency will certainly have weight related problems such as unexplained weight gain - even on a calorie controlled diet - or swings of gains and losses of body mass.

In addition, those with a zinc deficiency are likely to feel sluggish and tired. Therefore, their ability and motivation to exercise is impaired.

Since zinc deficiency is rife in society it is worth looking at the impact of zinc on weight and the underlying reasons why it might aid weight loss.

Zinc is essential for the smooth running of the thyroid gland. It is needed to produce thyroid stimulating hormone. The latter, if in short supply, results in low levels of T4 and T3. These hormones help regulate the body's metabolism turning food into energy. Without the proper synthesis of these hormones not only will weight gain occur but the person who lacks these thyroid hormones will feel cold and tired.

Zinc supplements help to increase the weight loss of those on a calorie restricted diets. In a study, calorie reduction of 300Kj was undertaken by individuals supplemented with 30mg of zinc. The control group did not receive any supplementary zinc. This regime was followed for 15 weeks.

After 15 weeks there was a significant reduction of body weight, BMI, waist circumference in the zinc supplemented group. In addition, it was found that there were lower levels of C-reactive protein, insulin resistance and appetite score.

Therefore, zinc appears to tackle obesity from different angles. Firstly, it helps correct any deficiency which might impact the metabolic rate. Secondly, it tackles insulin resistance enabling food to be used as an energy source instead of being used for fat storage. Thirdly, it aids appetite reduction and fourthly it helps tackle inflammation.

Many comorbid conditions occur alongside obesity and metabolic syndrome. They are all associated with zinc deficiency. There are a number of skin reactions, including psoriasis, that may be due to insufficient zinc in the diet. Delayed wound healing, decline of reproductive capacity, mental lethargy, depression, and susceptibility to Alzheimer's Disease are also included.

Oxidative stress underlies the molecular mechanisms responsible for the development of many inflammatory diseases like atherosclerosis, diabetes mellitus, rheumatoid arthritis as well as neurodegenerative disorders. The cellular antioxidant system proves insufficient to remove the reactive oxygen species which damage cells and create inflammation in this process.

The regulatory function of zinc cannot be underestimated. It is essential to the structure and function of nearly 3000 macromolecules and over 300 enzymes.

What may you be asking has this to do with EDS? Is there a link?

Zinc is not only connected with weight gain but it is responsible for making macromolecules from amino acids.

Macromolecules are very large molecules such as proteins made from amino acids. One of these macromolecules just happens to be collagen, the main protein found in connective tissue. Zinc deficiency may well contribute to the poor formation of connective tissue found in those with EDS.

Common macromolecules, monomers and some end products are:

MACROMOLECULE	MONOMERS (the building blocks)	END PRODUCT
protein	Amino acids	Protein – many types such as keratin for hair and collagen for connective tissue, enzymes and antibodies.
Nucleic acids	Nucleotides	RNA and DNA
Lipids	Fatty acids	Fats, sterols, waxes and oils

The importance of having adequate daily amounts of zinc cannot be underestimated. Zinc has been described as the element with a minor plasma pool and a rapid turnover.

There are certain groups of individuals that are more susceptible to zinc deficiency. These include:

- Diabetics
- Cancer patients
- Those with liver disease
- Those on a high plant diet as the phytates in plants bind to zinc
- Those on high copper or high iron diets
- Those who are on a calorie reducing diet
- Those who are under stress
- The elderly
- Breast fed babies
- Pregnant women
- Alcoholism
- Those with malabsorption problems of the digestive tract such as Crohn's disease.

Sources of zinc include:

- Oysters (very high in zinc) 3 ounces provides 673% of the daily value
- Beef – 3 ounces provide 65% of your daily requirements
- Beef patty – 3 ounces provides 64% of your daily requirement
- Baked beans – half a cup provides 26% of your daily requirement.

The benefits of zinc for metabolic syndrome and its related comorbidities cannot be understated.

The Daily Requirement of Zinc has been placed at'

Men – 11g

Women 8mg

However, for short periods of no greater than a month, upwards of this amount may be used to aid the processes which counteract metabolic syndrome. Any longer and you raise the risk of iron and copper depletion which carry their own risk of deficiency diseases.

Boron

Boron is a trace mineral that has many important functions in the body that are relevant to metabolic syndrome. While boron is generally associated with the health of bone it is essential for wound healing which is often delayed in those with metabolic syndrome.

Further, boron is required for the optimum use of hormones such as oestrogen and testosterone. It is able to increase oestrogen in post-menopausal women and healthy men. Oestrogen is important when looking at potential reasons for weight gain because low levels may contribute to abdominal weight gain.

Boron enhances magnesium and vitamin D absorption and also helps reduce inflammatory markers such as C-reactive protein and tumour necrosis factor (TNF-α).

C-reactive protein is a substance produced by the liver in response to inflammation. The blood test for C-reactive protein is a common one. While it tests for levels of inflammation it cannot indicate the cause of the inflammation. However, as inflammation is rife in those with obesity, it is a good test in that it alerts you to this underlying problem and the need to address it.

TNF-α is also a marker of inflammation. It helps to coordinate the inflammatory process. Sometimes, levels of TNF may get out of control. When it does symptoms may include:

- Low blood pressure

- Loss of appetite

- Redness and swelling at the site of injury

- Fever and muscle aches and pains

There is also an association between TNF-α and insulin resistance responsible for diabetes type. It is a bit of a catch 22 situation because insulin resistance leads to obesity and obesity promotes the generation of more TNF-α which in turn leads to greater insulin resistance. TNF is released by many cells including:

- Macrophages

- T cells

- Fibroblasts

- Dendritic cells

- Fat cells

In particular, TNF is highly likely to affect cells that line blood vessels creating inflammation and laying down an environment for plaques which block blood flow.

Vascular problems that ensue cause angiogenesis (the formation of new blood vessels) which is found in conditions like lymphoedema, obesity and cancer.

TNF may also be responsible for intestinal problems such as irritable bowel syndrome and the inflammatory bowel diseases such as Crohn's disease. It does this by stimulating effector T cells and macrophages. When these cells are stimulated they produce more inflammatory substances and resist programmed cell death, a process known as apoptosis. Apoptosis is required to eliminate cancerous cells.

There are many factors that increase TNF and these include but are not limited to:

- A lack of exercise but **excessive** exercise would increase TNF.

- Obesity

- High glucose levels

- A high fat diet

- Smoking and alcohol

- Deficiencies of choline, magnesium, zinc, chromium and vitamin D.

Finally, boron has a suppressive role on adiopogenic differentiation. What does this mean? Basically, pre fat cells develop into mature ones during this process of differentiation and is to be avoided if we are serious about losing weight. Boron prevents this maturation of pre fat cells into mature ones.

Boron can be taken up to 20mg daily but the normal supplemented dose is 3 mg. it is better to keep to the lower end of the dosage recommendations if you are using it just as a preventative. Boron, in very high doses, can actually cause weight gain and hair loss. In smaller doses its main function appears to be optimising the function of other vital nutrients and suppressing weight gain.

Good sources of boron are:

- Dried beans
- Milk
- Potatoes
- Coffee
- Apples
- Brazil nuts

As you can see a deficiency of nutrients that are only required in minute quantities can cause problems with unwanted weight gain. I am really quite concerned that the majority of the medical profession believe that weight gain can only be a result of too many calories in and not enough expended. There are many variables that need to be considered first especially in conditions like EDS.

Conditions can be difficult to live without the negative judgement of others

Brown fat, white fat – what's serotonin got to do with it?

All fat is not equal when it comes to burning calories. The fact that fat burns any calories may come as a surprise to some. After all, we can understand that we store fat but not that it burns calories but while white fat builds up in obesity, brown fat produces an important protein that helps to promote energy to generate heat. Therefore, it seems wise to take a closer look at these two types of fat.

White fat is found in the subcutaneous region, that is just under the skin. It provides the padding we need so that we do not injure ourselves and also provides insulation in cold weather. This type of fat is also the visceral fat, found around organs which pumps out inflammatory chemicals and is likely to raise your blood pressure as well as deposit itself in that well known apple shape found in metabolic syndrome.

Brown fat is found in deposits around the kidneys, along the spinal cord and between the shoulder blades. It consists of many lipid droplets. There is far less brown fat than white fat in obese people and brown fat does not build up in obese people.

Research has shown that white fat is linked with certain branched chain and aromatic amino acids.

The branched chain amino acids are:

- Leucine
- Isoleucine
- Valine

The aromatic amino acids are:

- Phenylalanine
- Tyrosine

These amino acids when eaten have been closely related to type 2 diabetes, insulin resistance, obesity and future diabetes.

As these amino acids are so important to the progression of diabetes the main sources of these are tabulated below.

Table showing the amino acids associated with obesity and their main sources

Amino acids	Food sources
Leucine	Dairy, soy, beans and legumes
Isoleucine	Beef, chicken, pork, tuna, dairy, lentils and beans[13]
Valine	Soy, cheese, peanuts, mushrooms, whole grains, vegetables
Phenylalanine	Dairy, meat, poultry, soy, beans, nuts and fish
tyrosine	Poultry, fish, peanuts, nuts, bananas, dairy, lima beans pumpkin and sesame seeds

Now as you can see most of the foods that can contribute to obesity are the high protein foods – those very foods you are told to eat because if you keep up the high protein foods and cut out fat/and or/ carbohydrates then you will lose weight.

---

[13] https://www.myfooddata.com/articles/high-isoleucine-foods.php#isoleucine-food-list

This may happen for some individuals - depending on genetics and other factors - but others will just find that they want to binge on something sweet when they are on a high protein, low carbohydrate/fat diet.

There is real science why this is so and why many people on a high protein diet cannot lose weight. It is all to do with brown fat

Brown fat produces a protein called SLC25A44 which for simplicity sake I am just going to call brown fat protein. It has a special function in that it brings the branched chain amino acids into the mitochondria, where they are used to provide energy and generate heat. When this process is blocked, studies in mice have shown that higher serum levels of branched chain amino acids result in obesity and signs of diabetes.

The lack of serotonin blocks this process for serotonin enhances the function of brown fat which is to specifically break down blood sugar and fat molecules.

Serotonin is found in carbohydrates and sugary foods. Its parent amino acid is tryptophan an amino acid which has the largest molecules of any amino acid.

When it tries to compete with other amino acids to cross the blood brain barrier, it gets left behind. It really needs a little carbohydrate to help it to accomplish this task.

Tryptophan can follow one of two pathways. It can go down the kyurenic acid pathway. Kyurenic acid inhibits colon cancer proliferation. Alternatively, it can become part of central serotonin which increases energy expenditure by enhancing the sympathetic drive to brown adipose tissue.

Serotonin is the happiness hormone. It stops you feeling anxious and depressed. It can be seen that too little carbohydrate to protein in the diet just promotes a build-up of branched chain amino acids leading to obesity, diabetes and metabolic syndrome.

Tryptophan requires the enzyme tryptophan hydroxylase to convert it to serotonin.

This enzyme is dependent on oxygen and a substance called tetrahydrobiopterin for regulation. Therefore, they are cofactors and vital for the conversion of tryptophan to its intermediate – 5 htp – to serotonin.

Nutrients which support the production of tetrahydrobiopterin are:

- Vitamin C
- Curcumin
- Methyl folate

Vitamin C is found in fresh fruit and vegetables. It is a water soluble vitamin and cannot be stored in the body as the fat soluble vitamins A, D, E and K can, therefore it is better that fresh fruit and vegetables are eaten every day. It is easily destroyed by sunlight and heat so cook any vegetables lightly.

Curcumin is a bright yellow compound produced by the Curcuma longa plant found in turmeric which is used in curries. It is better known as a natural compound which has anti-viral activity. Investigations showed that it had efficacy against influenza A as well as a wide range of other.

Methyl folate is the active form of folic acid. It is also referred to as vitamin B9. This is an important vitamin which aids the conversion of homocysteine (a harmful amino acid) back into the harmless methionine.

There are many good sources of methyl folate which include:

- Dark green leafy vegetables especially spinach and Brussels sprouts.
- liver
- Fruit
- Legumes
- Seafood
- Eggs
- Dairy products
- Meat
- grains

Many people who have been on a high protein diet for a long time and have failed to lose weight should try supplementing their diet with tryptophan 500mg –or 5htp - which is obtainable as a supplement (must be taken without other forms of protein but with a little carbohydrate for it to be absorbed). Alternatively, they could try substituting some of their protein for a little carbohydrate.

In a nutshell

SEROTONIN PERSUADES BROWN FAT TO BURN UP THE AMINO ACIDS WHICH CONTRIBUTE TO OBESITY, METABOLIC SYNDROME AND DIABETES

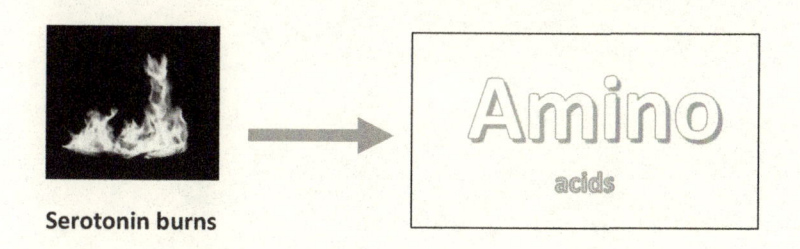

Serotonin burns → Amino acids

SEROTONIN IS FORMED FROM TRYPTOPHAN WHICH IS A LARGE AMINO ACID.

TRYPTOPHAN IS SO BIG THAT IT IS UNABLE TO COMPETE WITH OTHER SMALLER AMINO ACIDS TO CROSS THE BLOOD BRAIN BARRIER ON A TRANSPORTER. THEREFORE, IT IS BETTER TO BE TAKEN BY ITSELF WITH A LITTLE CARBOHYDRATE.

Or

YOU CAN SUPPLEMENT WITH 5HTP WHICH IS THE INTERMEDIARY PRODUCT FORMED OF TRYPTOPHAN AND SEROTONIN.

Tryptophan is in most **high**-protein **foods**, including wheat germ, cottage cheese, chicken, and turkey.

The final word

Early childhood photographs show genu curvatum – a backwards bending of my knees. I could do the splits with ease and my party piece involved touching my thumb on the same side wrist.

As I grew up joint pain became a daily companion. I suffered repeated sprains and tendonitis, jaw subluxations, fatigue, repeated and crippling bouts of sciatica, soft tissue injury and many other symptoms of EDS.

When I was 25 years old I began to suffer from gastroparesis. Later I had gastro-oesophageal reflux disorder and, of course, the biggy – the splitting of the connective tissue between abdominal tissues leaving a 15cm gap.

I had allergies and angioedema.

I had the typical scarring pattern of those with EDS.

I bruised easily

I had MCAD and PoTS

Anxiety (not surprisingly)

My repeat prescriptions were growing by the minute but yet, still no diagnosis.

I found my best ally was the camera on my smartphone which showed without a doubt that my angieoedema, urticaria, among other symptoms was very real.

I had a family history – the hypermobility undoubtedly came from the maternal side but there is evidence of a connective tissue disorder on my father's side too.

I am thankful that my skills and abilities helped me not only research my symptoms but also provide a response, through diet to alleviate my symptoms.

Most people consider that EDS is a chronic and degenerative condition. While I will always have a genetic potential to EDS, I can categorically state that my condition has continued to improve and barely impacts my life now.

This is a lifelong condition and I am all too aware that should I let my diet slip, then I would likely return to the days when this condition ruled my life, entirely.

I have come to understand how medication has little to offer EDS and can often worsen the condition than improve it.

It really is important to consider that some of the side effects of taking medication may not be reversible once that medication is stopped.

Food is a medicine. There are many good steroid substitutes, for example, but without the side effects of steroids which thin skin and can worsen all the symptoms of EDS.

Do not let your condition master you. Master your condition.

Other books by this author include:

- The EDS and Hypermobility Syndrome Diet
- Alleviating Symptoms of EDS
- Gastroparesis
- The EDS recipe book
- The Lipoedema Diet
- The Lymphoedema Diet: reverse and repair lymphatic damage

For the full range visit the author website on

https://www.amazon.co.uk/-/e/B07BPQZ5CD

https://www.amazon.com/-/e/B07BPQZ5CD

Twitter Lynne D M Noble @ ldmn53

A percentage of the royalties from the sale of these books are donated to charity, like the Exodus Project below,

The Exodus Project

My first introduction to the far reaching impact of The Exodus Project occurred when I was travelling around Cawthorne in one of their buses, visiting gardens. A young lad was happily munching on a sandwich. He looked up briefly, pointed to the driver and said,' He's my second dad, he is,' then he returned to his sandwich without further comment

Such remarks are often very telling and so I arranged to meet Jackie Peel and Martin Sawdon, at the charity's premises in Barnsley. They set up the Exodus Project 20 years ago. They moved into their current premises – a redundant Methodist church - in 2010.

Both Jackie and Martin have been youth workers in their church. Martin worked in housing for the homeless in addition to working in learning disabilities services in institutional settings.

The work that the Exodus Project undertakes is of paramount importance to the communities it serves. These were former mining communities which became disadvantaged after pit-closures. Currently about 400 children attend mid-week activities from Monday to Thursday inclusive. These activities include dance, drama, craft, music, sports and games. In addition, there are weekend camps, cycle treks, outward bound activities, bowling and swimming. The children are taught valuable life skills including how to cook and bake. It is all about teaching children how to fulfil their potential and learn skills they will be able to pass onto the next generation.

The grounds, once overgrown, have been turned into a play- and camping - ground. A miniature railway is in the process of being installed.

Martin and Jackie have developed a unique model in that The Exodus Project goes beyond dispensing services. They are keen to build up relationships with the whole family and not just the child that attends the mid- week clubs. In addition, once children have reached the age of fourteen, they are invited to help out with the younger groups as junior volunteers. Once they reach the age of eighteen, they become adult volunteers. This model provides a constant supply of help from individuals who have benefitted already from attending such groups.

The building is large and inviting. It is decorated with bold colours and has comfy seating. It is a real home from home; a haven for families who have been disadvantaged by the closure of the life force of its community.

Martin and Jackie have clear ideas about how they wish to develop the Exodus Project but the lottery funding which they benefitted from is no longer available. Sadly, they have had to close two of their clubs due to lack of funding. This decision wasn't taken lightly. They do have two charity shops which raises some money and they obtain some funding from outside organisations for the use of their facilities. However, this is clearly not enough to keep their clubs, weekend activities and building going to cater for the ever growing number of children who are benefitting from the work being undertaken here. Neither does it allow for future development.

Exodus do have a Just Giving page which can be found here if you wish to help further their work https://www.justgiving.com/exodus

In addition, you can keep up with activities on their Facebook page here

https://www.facebook.com/search/top/?q=the%20exodus%20project%20barnsley&epa=SEARCH_BOX

If anyone wishes undertake an event like The Three Peaks - or run a marathon to raise funds for Exodus - then

Martin or Jackie would be pleased to hear from you. This will enable their vital work in the community to continue. Contact them through their website to be found on www.exodusproject.org.uk.

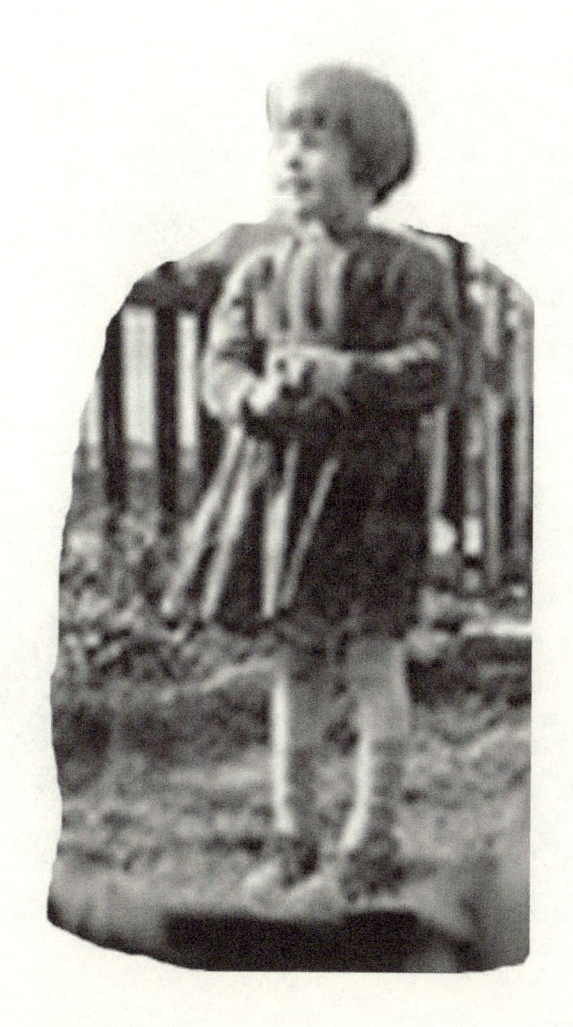

Author as a young girl

Note backward curve of left leg – genu curvatum

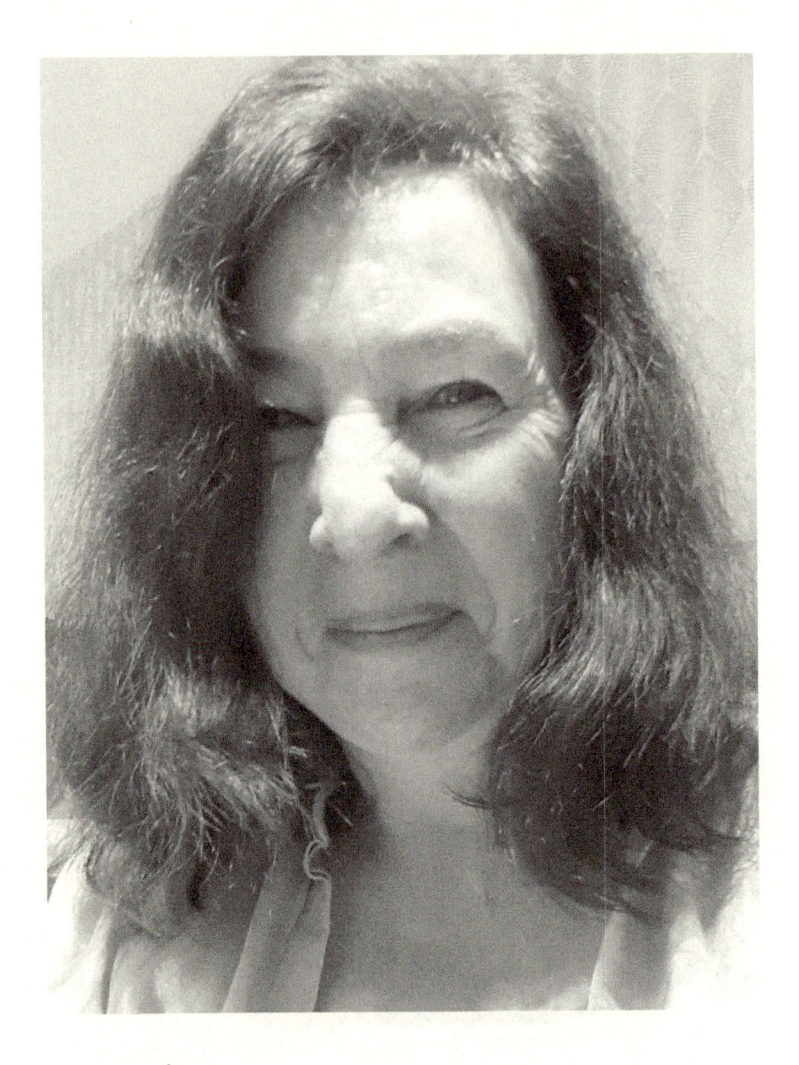

Lynne today

Made in the USA
Middletown, DE
26 June 2024